The Running Life

"Whether you are an experienced runner, a novice, or even a non-runner this compilation of articles will inspire."

Amby Burfoot, Editor at Large, *Runner's World Magazine* and 1968 Boston Marathon winner.

The Running Life

Wisdom and Observations from a Lifetime of Running

Donald Buraglio and Michael Dove

iUniverse, Inc.
New York Bloomington

The Running Life

Wisdom and Observations from a Lifetime of Running

iUniverse books may be ordered through booksellers or by contacting:

iUniverse
1663 Liberty Drive
Bloomington, IN 47403
www.iuniverse.com
1-800-Authors (1-800-288-4677)

ISBN: 978-1-4502-2169-6 (pbk)
ISBN: 978-1-4502-2170-2 (ebk)

Printed in the United States of America
iUniverse rev. date: 9/20/2010

TO OUR WIVES AND FAMILIES FOR
THEIR INSPIRATION, LOVE, AND

MOST IMPORTANTLY FOR THEIR PATIENCE

Table of Contents

Preface

The book you are holding is a sampling of columns from The Running Life, which appears every other week in the *Monterey County Herald*. Our columns run the gamut from instructional articles and training advice to public health issues and human interest stories, along with some light-hearted observations and occasional nonsense. They are intended for dedicated runners as well as those who've never laced up a pair of trainers. Above all else, they reflect our experiences and insights from a combined fifty years of running. We hope you enjoy our perspective and that it encourages you, if you don't already participate, to give our wonderful sport a try.

In this collection, columns are not presented in chronological order as they appeared in the newspaper; rather, they have been organized in categories based on subject matter. They don't need to be read from start to finish; you'll get just as much benefit reading in any order you choose. Jump in anyplace that looks interesting, and come back to the others another time.

Our goals in starting a newspaper column were to promote the sport of running in Monterey County, be an informative resource for runners, and hopefully make some people smile along the way. At first we feared that we'd run out of things to write about - but the more we kept running and observing, the more we realized that column material is never hard to find. Once the legs start moving, the creative process springs to life; we're not sure why or how this happens, but we're eternally grateful that it does.

We are extremely lucky to live in Monterey County, California, a beautiful geographic area that is also home to the Big Sur International Marathon and Big Sur Half Marathon. This book contains a special section of articles about each of those races, both because we've written about them for years, and because they hold a special place in our hearts. We would encourage anybody to visit and enjoy our majestic natural surroundings while taking part in our local world-class events.

Finally, we are particularly proud of programs we have started to encourage children and adults to start running. These are the Just Run program for children and Take 5 to Run for everyone. The fight against childhood obesity is a pet crusade of ours, and we urge you to start a Just Run program in your area. You'll find details about both of these programs in the pages ahead.

If you would like to follow us in the future, current columns are posted on the *Monterey Herald* website (www.montereyherald.com). You can also find us on Donald's Running and Rambling website at www.runningandrambling.com.

Thank you very much for your support. We hope you enjoy reading the articles as much as we enjoyed writing them.

Donald Buraglio and Michael Dove

Monterey County, California.

Introduction: Don't Run!

It's the first week of January, and you're probably overwhelmed with hearing New Year's resolutions. After all, nearly everybody spends this time of year blathering endlessly about how things will be different from now on, and how their lives will improve.

It's also the time when many people decide to start running to get in shape. While we think this is a noble goal, we're not going to preach to you about all the benefits of running – at least not right now.

Today we're doing the opposite. If you are one of those who have resolved to start running, listen closely. You think you want to be a runner? Sure, everyone wants to lose weight, feel better, and live longer – but have you ever considered that maybe the running life *isn't* all it's cracked up to be?

In some ways, being overweight and out of shape actually has its advantages. Once you decide to become a runner, there are plenty of drawbacks you'll need to deal with on an almost daily basis.

For instance, we hope you don't have any hang-ups about how you look in public. Once you step out the door and onto the road, there's a good chance that your neighbors, your friends, your customers or even your boss will see you. Are you comfortable being seen with unkempt hair, a snotty nose, no makeup, wearing shorts or tights, and sweating profusely from every pore? Then go ahead and lace up those shoes.

The risk of public dishevelment doesn't stop when your run ends, either. You know the one parent at school who always shows up wearing sweatpants, looking frazzled and unshowered when dropping the kids off in the morning, or the co-worker who always appears flushed and somewhat smelly during an afternoon meeting at work? If you're a runner, that person is *you*. Welcome to our club.

If you start telling people you're a runner, be forewarned that you'll have to answer for it seemingly forever. We can't count the number of conversations at social gatherings that have started with "So, are you still running?" or "How far did you run today?"

If you're consistent with your running, you'll always have a satisfactory answer. But heaven forbid you ever fall off the wagon, for everyone will know within 30 seconds of talking to you.

(Actually, we're curious as to why runners are always greeted like that. Do people talk to alcoholics or gamblers this way: "So, are you still drinking?" or "How much money did you squander this weekend?" Not that we're addicted to running. We could stop at any time. Besides, we're not harming anyone else. Let's just move on…)

Do you like eating at McDonald's or Burger King? If so, get your fill before you become a runner, because once you start running consistently, your body develops an aversion to many kinds of fast food. Are you sure you want to give up those Whoppers, curly fries and bacon croissants?

We've heard great things about fast food joints. Combo meals are supposedly pretty popular, and we've always wanted to say, "Super size me!!" to somebody. Plus, they still give away toys with some meals, don't they? Unfortunately, neither one of us has eaten in a fast food place for several years, so we miss out on all that fun.

Are you a bargain shopper? Do you like getting your money's worth? Maybe you should reconsider the whole idea of losing weight. Think of it like this: say you're buying a pair of jeans for $40. The pants with the 42-inch waistlines usually cost the same price as the 32-inch waists, right?

So if you have a 32-inch waist, you're getting 10 inches less material than the guy who buys the 42s for the same price. In other words, you're getting ripped off every time you buy clothes. Runners have suffered this kind of senseless waist-size discrimination for years, and look forward to a glorious day when we receive a discount for the lower quantity of material used. We have a dream!

Not to mention, if you start running and lose a lot of weight, you'll need to prepare for the expense of buying a new wardrobe.

Finally, we should address the popular notion that runners live longer than non-runners. OK, technically, yes, that's a proven fact. But many of those "extra" hours are spent doing the exercise that's supposedly buying you more time.

Let's say you exercise for an hour a day for 30 years – that's almost 11,000 total hours spent exercising. There are 8,760 hours in a year. So if running helps delay your fatal heart attack by only three years, you're really only gaining half of that amount of time for doing non-running stuff.

Yes, we're exaggerating a bit here, as runners typically live many years longer than sedentary people, and would therefore gain a great deal of extra time to spend with grandkids or walking on the beach. However, runners also tend to jeopardize their lives at a slightly higher rate than the general public, so they have to be extra careful.

Think of it this way: If you never go in the ocean, you'll never get eaten by a shark - but the more times you go swimming, the greater your chances become. This is how runners consider predators like buses and ignorant drivers. So if you become a runner, you'll be healthy enough to live longer, but there's also a better-than-average chance that you'll get run over by a garbage truck someday.

In that regard, it's clearly much safer to stay inside with your butt parked on the couch.

Running obviously isn't for sissies. So consider all these drawbacks before you invest too much time and effort in this habit of ours. Don't say we didn't warn you.

And what if you still want to be a runner? Congratulations – we think it's the best resolution you could ever make.

Now keep reading.

MOTIVATION AND INSPIRATION

"The wizard told them, 'I didn't give you anything that you didn't already have inside you. It just took you 26.2 miles to find it.'"

"Seek out your own valley of love and delight. Be thankful for your ability to run, and take pleasure in the fact that you are able to do it. Enjoy every mile of the journey, because we never know when we may be in the homestretch. Really, these should be the easy things to do."

You Had a Bad Day

Wait! Don't tell us – you make a resolution each New Year to lose weight and get healthy. And then you can barely get to the middle of January before it becomes an enormous struggle.

Everybody sabotages their fitness plans from time to time – even your local running columnists. So we're not going to beat you over the head with all the reasons you should be running.

Instead, we're going to take you through a typical day, and show you just how many opportunities there are to screw things up. Here's a small sampling of the ways you can have a bad day by neglecting your fitness plan over the course of 24 hours:

Last night, you ambitiously set your alarm 30 minutes early in order to exercise before your workday. But when the alarm goes off, the bed feels so warm and comfortable that you hit the snooze button to linger a bit longer. 10 minutes later, you do the same thing again; and later on, once more. So much for your morning exercise.

As you shower, you tell yourself that you'll compensate by hitting the gym at lunchtime, so you pack a duffel bag with workout clothes and figure you're still right on track with your training program.

You're running a bit behind, and you really aren't too hungry, so you hurry out the door without eating breakfast. But you're not fully alert yet, so you swing by Starbucks for a little pick-me-up. You received a gift card for Christmas, so it's not like you're spending real money.

You order a grande caramel macchiato and a big cranberry muffin. It's fine, because you skipped breakfast – and now you're at the top of your game.

Arriving at work, you park as close as possible to the building and take the elevator up to the 2nd floor. You stow your duffel bag in the corner before sitting down at your computer to catch up on e-mail. 90 minutes later, your office neighbor comes by with leftover Christmas cookies that his spouse made. (He's getting rid of them because he resolved to eat healthier this year.)

You smell the cookies and realize how hungry you are. So you grab a few cookies, which is OK because they're little ones, and because you didn't eat breakfast. You eat one of them now, and put the others on your desk to save for the afternoon. 10 minutes later, those are gone as well.

At 11:30 your co-workers stop by to invite you out to lunch with them. You stare at your duffel bag for about 2 seconds then agree to go along. It's OK, because you might be able to quit work a bit early and go for a quick run before going home. You crowd onto the elevator with your co-workers and head down to the car.

You go to your favorite restaurant and order a big meal, since you're still catching up from breakfast. It's OK to eat big though, because you've started a fitness program, and you'll burn all those calories off soon enough.

During meetings and phone calls after lunch, you gradually feel your energy level wavering. At 3:00 it seems like a good time to visit your co-worker who always keeps a bowl full of Reese's mini peanut butter cups at his desk. It's OK, because those are your favorite candy.

You talk to him a bit and idly eat 3 minis, then decide to grab a couple more as you head back to your desk, which is OK, since they're minis. You sit back down with renewed energy, a smile on your face, and a bit of chocolate on your cheek.

You finish the work day and make it all the way to your car before you realize that you left the duffel bag in your office. At this point, it's a total hassle to go back inside to get it, since you'd have to wait for the elevator, then say goodnight to everyone all over again. Besides, you figure that traffic is crazy, so you don't really have any extra time to work out. It's OK, because you'll have three chances to exercise tomorrow.

On your way home, you call your family, and decide that it would be a lot easier to go out for dinner instead of cooking tonight – so you meet them at the pizza parlor.

You have 3 pieces of pepperoni pizza, 2 pieces of garlic bread and a glass of red wine. It's OK, because garlic and wine are good for your heart, and because you're going to skip the spumoni dessert.

At home you spend two hours sitting on the couch, catching up on TV and reviewing the newspaper and magazine articles about exercise that you've been collecting.

As you climb into bed, you try to get friendly with your spouse, but she complains that you smell like garlic. So you go into the kitchen and have a big bowl of ice cream. It's OK, because ice cream is your comfort food – and besides, you're going to set your alarm early tomorrow to start exercising.

So you had a bad day. These things happen to all of us. The trick is to make sure it doesn't become a cycle that repeats itself day after day.

Bad days don't become perfect ones overnight, and fitness doesn't happen immediately. Changes are small, and gradual, and usually happen one at a time. But if you dedicate yourself to achieving them, you'll gradually make big improvements over the course of the year.

If you've made a resolution to get in shape, we hope that your new fitness program is filled with many more good days than bad ones.

Runners' Goals for a New Year

Sedentary people typically make fitness resolutions in early January – and then by February, all bets are off. This isn't surprising, as studies have shown that it's actually easier to kick a smoking or drug habit than it is to start and maintain a fitness program.

Runners, on the other hand, tend to be fairly goal-oriented and disciplined, with a passion for the sport (as opposed to, say, a StairMaster – does anyone honestly get passionate about that?) and a solid work ethic, so there's no limit to what a determined runner can do.

Sometimes, however, even experienced runners can use some suggestions. The following goals range from very basic to seemingly crazy. Our point is this: the particular goal you have doesn't really matter. What's important is that you are progressing and challenging your current level of fitness. Anything you do tomorrow that is more than you have been doing lately is wonderful. Consider these options:

Run one mile continuously. The basic unit of measurement for distance running is a perfect tangible goal for someone who is just starting a running program. Build up to this by alternating walk/run intervals, and gradually decrease the amount of time spent walking. Don't worry at first about how long the mile takes you- save that for later (see below).

Run a sub-*x* minute mile. A generation ago, the mile was the most glamorous event in sports. Though its popularity has since declined, it remains the ultimate test of combined stamina and power. However, unless they've been in the military, most runners have no idea what their best mile time is. So go to a track and find out, and then try to improve enough to go under the closest round minute. (Note- although tracks are now measured in meters, most all-weather tracks still have markings for the one-mile start and finish.)

Run a 5K. This is a great entry-level goal for two reasons: 1) The distance is significant enough (3.1 miles) to require a bit of advance preparation, and 2) The best way to run 5K is in a race, which is like a public declaration of your new fitness activity. Local 5Ks are great places to meet fellow runners and stay motivated to keep training.

Find your best 10K time. This is the benchmark standard for the vast majority of road racers. Start running with any new group and it may only be a matter of minutes before someone asks about your best 10K time. So why not find out? Find a race to enter, and jump in. Remember to race cautiously. It's very easy to get carried away and start too fast before crashing miserably after the halfway point. In many ways, the 10K is the most difficult distance running event - because unlike a marathon, people usually try to run as fast as they can, and unlike a 5K, it's an extremely long distance to run at maximal effort.

Run a sub-50, or sub-40-minute 10K. It's human nature that once you find your best 10K time, you would want to improve it. The 10K has well-known landmark times that runners often strive to accomplish. A 50-minute 10K requires an average pace of 8:03 per mile, and sub-40 requires 6:27 miles.

Break your age in a 10K. For example, if you are 43 years old, try to run a sub-43 minute 10K. The younger you are, the more impressive this feat is. Olympic-caliber runners can do it in their late 20s, top amateur runners in their early-to-mid 30s, and good recreational runners in their 40s.

Run a half marathon. The distance requires fairly dedicated training, but not to the extreme degree that marathon training demands. Autumn is a popular season for half marathons; build up your training through the spring and summer, and be ready for race day in the fall.

Run a marathon. Most runners see this as the ultimate challenge. The marathon certainly has the most mystique of any distance race, and its siren call beckons an increasing number of runners every year. Many people attempt to run the marathon just to know the experience. Once they finish, some are content to retire, while others become addicted to the euphoric feeling this race offers. Fortunately for us, one of the best marathons in North America - the Big Sur International - is right in our backyard. However, there are many excellent marathons in scenic locations and at various times of the year throughout the United States.

Run a sub-3 or sub-4 hour marathon. Don't worry about how long your first marathon takes; just pace yourself to finish and feel (relatively) good at the end. Once you have one or two finishes under your belt, then strive for a target time. Just as 1-minute intervals are benchmarks for the mile, 1-hour intervals are milestones for the marathon. Tell a runner that you're a sub-3-hour marathoner and he'll know that you're fast. Tell your training group that you want to break 4 hours, and they'll help you practice the necessary pace during your training runs. For the record, a sub-3 marathon is 6:52/mile; sub-4 is 9:10/mile.

Do an ultramarathon. If you've done several marathons and are looking for a more challenging endurance event, ultras may be for you. The typical distances are 50K, 50-mile, and 100-mile. Training for a 50K (31 miles) is actually not much harder than a marathon. Most ultras are on trails and dirt roads, through scenic wilderness areas, and feature hills that are steeper and longer than any road race you'll ever see.

Clearly, there is a multitude of new challenges to set for yourself in the coming year. Choose wisely, and start training!

The 10,000 Hour Rule

Most runners probably don't think they have much in common with the likes of Mozart, The Beatles, or Bill Gates. However, according to Malcolm Gladwell, we have more in common than we ever realized.

Gladwell is the author of *Outliers: The Story of Success,* which enjoyed a long tenure atop bestseller lists nationwide. In the book, he analyzes countless factors – many of them unknown to the people they most impact – that determine why some people enjoy abundant success in life, while others toil in frustration and obscurity.

One of his revelations is the "10,000 Hour Rule": in order to maximize any given talent, you need to spend approximately 10,000 hours practicing it. This rule partially dispels the myths of the child prodigy or the naturally gifted artist that many of us accept at face value.

For example, Bill Gates is widely considered a genius – but he also happened to have extraordinary access to cutting-edge technologies as far back as junior high school, and he spent nearly every night and weekend of his youth experimenting with computer programming. Mozart wrote symphonies at age 4, but the body of work he's recognized for was composed after he had spent another 10 years perfecting his craft. And by the time The Beatles burst onto the American scene, they had developed their songwriting and polished their musical chops in thousands of shows in various foreign nightclubs.

The 10,000 Hour Rule has implications for runners as well – in fact, veteran runners have used a variation of it for a long time, known in running circles as the 10-Year Rule. Basically, it says that runners will get gradually faster during their first 10 years, before their performances plateau for another 10 years, then decline steadily over the next 10 years.

It doesn't matter what distance you run, or what age you start at: whether you're 15 or 55, your best race times in any event will improve for up to 10 years if you train consistently. If you could somehow manage to run 1000 hours per year, you'd develop abilities on par with some of the greatest achievers of our age. Sure, natural talent also plays a role – but not nearly as much as most people attribute to it. (And yes, at first glance, training for 1000 hours per year – averaging 3 hours per day, every day – seems shocking. However, if you ask just about any Olympic athlete, they'd tell you this is consistent with their typical regimens. There's a reason why it's so hard to make it to the Olympics.)

Perhaps the most well-known novel about running is *Once a Runner* by John Parker. In one famous passage, the author ponders how somebody becomes a great runner: "What was the secret, they wanted to know … and not one of them was prepared to believe that it had not so much to do with chemicals and zippy mental tricks as with that most unprofound and sometimes heart-rending process of removing, molecule by molecule, the very tough rubber that comprised the bottoms of his training shoes."

In other words, there's no secret, and no trick. Do you want to be a better runner? Go for a run. Wake up the next day and do it again. Keep doing it until you wear out the bottoms of your shoes, then buy some new ones and start again. Repeat that process over and over until you've done it for 1,000 hours, then 2,000, then 10,000.

It's really quite a simple process. Sometimes we just need to be reminded.

Dorothy from Del Rey Oaks

This story may sound familiar; it's the story of a lady we know. For the sake of anonymity, we'll call her Dorothy, who lives in Del Rey Oaks, a small town near the Monterey Peninsula.

Dorothy was approaching middle age, had just been through a messy divorce, and her self-esteem was extremely low. She had gained weight over the years and felt depressed all the time. She had no close friends to talk to other than her dear Aunt Emily.

Her only enjoyment came from walking her little dog Bobo around the lake in the morning before work. She would sometimes get lost in thought on her walks, and gradually started walking longer and longer distances.

One morning during her walk, Bobo broke loose from his leash. Dorothy ran to chase him, and made it halfway around the lake before a jogger helped out by scooping Bobo up and waiting for Dorothy. Dorothy could barely thank the man because she was so winded from the running, but afterward she felt exhilarated from the chase.

The next day Dorothy and Bobo saw the man again. She didn't want to slow him down, so she tried jogging alongside him so they could talk. His name was Scott, and he worked as a night watchman. Scott said he wanted a better job, but his opportunities were limited because he dropped out of high school. He thought if he was only a little smarter, he could finish his education someday to advance his career.

Dorothy enjoyed the conversation and didn't even realize she had jogged for about 20 minutes.

Scott and Dorothy began jogging together other every other day. They even ventured out on the recreation trail toward Monterey. One morning on the trail they came across a runner who seemed injured because of his stiff-legged stride. Fortunately, he wasn't really hurt and he asked if he could run with them for a bit.

He said his name was Tim, but in high school, his track teammates called him "Tim the Man" because he used to be so fast. Tim explained that his joints occasionally felt stiff at the beginning of a run, but after he warmed up he would be fine. Dorothy noticed that he seemed to take in a lot of fluids when he ran.

Tim became a running partner of Scott and Dorothy. He had a sensitive side to him, and explained that he also had gone through a bad breakup. Sometimes he felt like his heart had been ripped right out of his body.

The group began meeting on weekends to run longer distances together. One Saturday, they ran all the way to Lover's Point in Pacific Grove and stopped to look at the view. Bobo walked over to a man sitting in the grass and the man started yelling profanities at the dog. Dorothy confronted the man, who apologized and began to cry.

His name was Leon, and he had just settled in Pacific Grove after living for a while in Africa. He said he had a job as a safari guide, but failed miserably after realizing that he was terrified of almost all animals – even little dogs. Leon had lashed out at Bobo so he wouldn't appear too cowardly.

Dorothy, Scott, and Tim asked Leon to join them on next weekend's run. The four became close friends and running partners.

One January morning, Dorothy showed up with entry blanks for the Big Sur Marathon at the end of April. Her three partners had the following reactions:

Scott said, "I'm not smart enough to train correctly."

Tim the Man said: "I don't know if my heart is strong enough to do it."

Leon said, "I'm scared that I might not finish."

Dorothy said, "I hear that the Chairman of the Board, Hugo Ferlito, has run all 21 Big Sur Marathons. He stands at the finish line and helps hand out medals. The guy's some kind of running wizard. We can probably learn something from him." Finally her partners agreed to enter the race.

Scott did some research and mapped out a training plan, even getting advice from some of those small, skinny runners he knew from the local running guild. He realized the group had to increase their training right away to have enough time to prepare.

They ran together for the next three months, and when the training miles got difficult, they came up with a mantra to help them continue: "Follow the hilly black road! Follow the hilly black road!"

Finally, marathon day arrived, and it was one of the worst weather days in Big Sur history. The wind seemed strong enough to make houses fly. It was like a tornado out there! Dorothy commented, "Bobo – We're not in Del Rey Oaks anymore." It looked to be a real witch of a day.

But Dorothy and her friends persevered and finished the race. Scott had a smart race strategy of running easy in the early miles. Tim used a heart rate monitor to ensure a solid effort throughout the race. Leon showed great courage to battle through "the wall" at mile 22.

They all finished with their hands in the air and big smiles on their faces. And Hugo Ferlito, the wonderful wizard they heard about, handed each of them a finisher's medal.

After the race, Dorothy realized that she had lost 25 pounds and regained her self esteem. Tim the Man felt like he was falling in love again. Scott returned to school, passed his high school equivalency exam, and enrolled in classes at the local junior college. Leon took a job working with sharks at the Monterey Bay Aquarium.

Later that summer, they saw Hugo the Wizard running on the rec trail. They all graciously thanked him for the gifts they received.

And the wizard told them, "I didn't give you anything that you didn't already have inside you. It just took you 26.2 miles to find it."

Donald Buraglio and Michael Dove

Simple Gifts

For most people, shoe purchases are the most cost-prohibitive aspect of running. Typical training shoes only last about 400-500 miles before needing replacement, which for most recreational runners works out to about two or three pairs annually. Marathon runners, however, are a different breed; we frequently run more than 75 miles per week, and it's not uncommon to burn through several pairs of shoes each year.

It's no wonder then that every time I (Donald) find myself at the running store shelling out for yet another pair of shoes, I think about one of my favorite runners of all time, Ethiopian Abebe Bikila, and how much money I could save by emulating him.

Bikila's story is legendary among marathoners, and even among casual sports fans of the 1960s. He was one of the greatest marathoners in history, and his Olympic triumphs foreshadowed the domination of distance running by East African nations that has lasted over 50 years.

Prior to his competitive running career, Bikila served as an imperial bodyguard for Emperor Haile Selassie. He had only run two previous marathons before lining up at the starting line of the 1960 Rome Olympics in nothing more than a pair of shorts and a singlet; he chose to race barefoot, as he did in his youth (typical of many East African children), and as was his custom while training in the hilly farmlands of his home country. He is best remembered as the solitary figure pulling away from the pack as darkness fell, traversing the torch-lit cobblestone streets of the ancient city on his approach to the stadium, on his way to winning the Olympic marathon with naked feet. In so doing, he became a personification of the noble simplicity of distance running.

Bikila found more success in the years that followed, and in 1964 became the first person to win back-to-back Olympic marathon gold medals - although this time, he wore shoes. Unfortunately, his triumphs couldn't protect him from heartache and tragedy, in both his running and his life. He dropped out of the 1968 Olympic marathon due to an injury. One year later he was involved in a car accident that left him paralyzed and no longer able to run through the fields he loved as a child. In 1973 he died from a brain hemorrhage at the age of 41.

Runners frequently get caught up in collecting more "stuff" that we feel is absolutely necessary to improve our performance. We lust after gear and gadgets that we're convinced we can't do without: technical apparel, GPS devices, nutritional supplements, heart-rate monitors, blister-proof socks, polarized sunglasses, computer software to analyze our training programs, rainproof jackets, moisture-wicking underwear, and so on. This is in addition to all of the technological advances that are found in our once-basic pair of running shoes.

It's enough to make us forget that one of the most beautiful aspects of running is its simplicity – and one of the greatest enemies of that intrinsic beauty is rampant materialism. Consequently, if we're too focused on our shoes and gadgets and gizmos, we lose sight of the greater benefits that running provides us.

The old Shaker hymn tells us, "It's a gift to be simple, it's a gift to be free/ It's a gift to come down where we ought to be/ When we find ourselves in the place just right/ We will be in the valley of love and delight." So what does it mean to be simple and free? Perhaps the best way to understand is to observe children playing.

For example, my 6-year-old recently ran a 60-meter dash at a local track meet. He didn't care about how fast he went, and he was oblivious to all the other kids who ran faster than he did. After finishing, he jumped in the air and started giving everybody high fives. My 3-year-old daughter takes endless pleasure in sprinting up and down the hallway of our house, for no other reason than to see how fast she can make her legs move. And my infant daughter has just learned to walk, inevitably beaming with delight and pride as she crosses the room with outstretched arms. My kids' happiness stems from an inherent love of activity, and the pure gratification of movement.

East African children know this as well; the difference is that many of them are able to retain that perspective well into adulthood. In western society, we seem to lose our youthful enthusiasm and simple delights as we grow up. Thankfully, running provides an opportunity to tap into those emotions anytime we like.

The trick is learning not to dwell on the superficial things that we think will help us run better or faster. I like to remind myself that Abebe Bikila trained without a watch, did his long training runs without drinking Gatorade, and won the Olympic marathon without shoes. I like to watch my kids run around without inhibition, delighting in their bodies and the basic abilities with which they were blessed.

That's not to say that all of us need to run barefoot - although I'm certainly not opposed to the idea - but we should rediscover our simple gifts in other ways. Leave your watch at home sometimes before you run. Savor the child-like joy of moving across the earth under your own power. Run barefoot in the grass. Stop and look at the view at the top of a hill, or gaze at the water in the stream you are crossing.

Seek out your own valley of love and delight. Be thankful for your ability to run, and take pleasure in the fact that you are able to do it. Enjoy every mile of the journey, because we never know when we may be in the homestretch. Really, these should be the easy things to do. You don't even need a pair of shoes.

Running Tweets

First, some disclosure: We're not on Twitter. We've never tweeted. We're pretty much outcasts in the brave new world of social media.

However, we were curious as to whether Twitter had any value when it comes to dispensing sage running advice – so we asked many of our best local runners and coaches to tell us how to be a better runner. We only gave them one rule: their answer had to follow Twitter rules and be 140 characters or less.

Here are our favorite responses from the experts …

Former Olympic marathoner Nelly Wright from Pacific Grove: "It is all about attitude. Be positive. Be a good sportsman. Be consistent. Be passionate. Don't let setbacks get you down. Have fun."

Professional triathlete Alexis Waddell from Seaside: "Set a goal. Write out the training plan. Follow through with your workouts; consistency plays a major role in becoming a better runner."

North County HS coach Gus took the team approach: "Everyone is a winner. Running takes work. Expect the best. The team/family concept overrides any individual achievement."

Chris, Hartnell College coach: "As you get older focus less on the mileage and go back to your youth and hit the track. Train like you did in high school and college."

Jeff from Marina was very specific: "Get fast! Mon. do 3 to 7 one mile repeats at 10K pace. Weds. do 16 one minute "pulls" at 5K pace. On Sat. a four to 10 mile tempo run at half marathon pace."

Jim from Salinas showed impressive versatility, as his answer qualified as both a tweet and a rhyme: "You want to run fast? Just get off your behind or you will place last!"

Matt, a former 2:14 marathoner from Salinas: "There are no secrets or shortcuts in this sport. Train hard, but be smart enough to listen to what your body is telling you. Don't let your ego get in the way."

Some local runners didn't even need the full 140 characters to dispense their wisdom …

Former Olympic marathoner and *Runner's World* Magazine runner of the year Maria Trujillo: "Run fast and work hard."

Patty Selbicky, former winner of the Big Sur Marathon: "Intervals, intervals, and more intervals…..and listen to Glynn."

Of course, we then went straight to her friend Glynn, who is the dean of local runners, with over 65 years of competitive running and coaching experience. His tweet? "Run Run Run!" It's kind of eloquent in its simplicity.

We were actually fairly surprised to discover some valuable lessons in these short bursts, and considered our Great Twitter Experiment a bona fide success. Each individual tweet is interesting on its own, and when we put all the recommendations together, an ideal overall strategy emerges:

1. Be positive and optimistic.
2. Be consistent in your training.
3. You have to be thoughtful and have a plan.
4. To be fast you have to practice running fast.
5. There are no secrets and there is no substitute for hard work.
6. Enjoy the process.

Sounds like great advice to us.

Go All-In

Without a doubt, poker is hot.

High-stakes tournaments are televised year-round on multiple networks, and it seems like everyone wants to try their luck and live like The Gambler. Heck, even rinky-dink, small-town newspapers often have a regular poker column to teach a novice player how to work his short stack into a huge pile. We're pretty sure those are poker terms.

The World Series of Poker (WSOP) in Las Vegas now awards $10 million to the winner of the main event. The WSOP is televised on ESPN, and it's a unique glance into the world of high-stakes gambling that the vast majority of us are too poor - the entry fee to the main event is $10,000 - or too terrified to enter.

WSOP contestants make for fascinating viewing; it's the biggest collection of geeks and oddballs this side of a Star Trek convention. Harvard PhDs compete with uneducated laborers, arithmatic whiz kids stare down vice peddlers, and fresh-off-the-boat immigrants play alongside old-school Texas oilmen.

There are high rollers, Jesus freaks, pregnant women, and LOTS of fat guys. If someone could invent smell-o-vision, we would even sense the cigar stench and the stale nachos and the B.O. (come to think of it, maybe we could do without smell-o-vision).

Knowing this, and considering that the tournament is televised on the world's largest sports programming network, a couple of questions beg to be asked: 1) Can poker legitimately be called a sport, or its players considered athletes? And more specifically as far as runners are concerned, 2) Are there any lessons that endurance athletes can learn by watching?

The answers may surprise you.

Question #1 is easy: no one would dare call card players athletes. Even casual observers can take one look and tell that these folks aren't exactly smoothie-after-a-workout types.

However, question #2 is more complex. The main event of the WSOP, a ruthless variety of poker called No-limit Texas Hold 'Em, does in fact have some parallels to running. One dramatic similarity is the most exciting aspect of the game, when players decide to "go all-in."

In the no-limit game, anyone can wager their entire stack of chips on any given hand. If you have a higher chip count, you can go all-in against a lower stack to intimidate them off a hand, further building your pile. If you go all-in with the low stack and lose the hand, you're out of the tournament.

You might think players would reserve such a gambit for only a few premium hands, but it's actually done all the time. Tournament rules require increasing chip bids for each hand, so the player who plays conservatively will slowly bleed his chips away before the ideal hand comes along. Thus, going all-in is a necessity, as players are unable to win large pots or knock other players out without this tactic.

Think of going all-in as running a race. It represents a time to push all of your chips onto the table, reveal your cards, and see who comes out on top.

In poker, the decision to go all-in is partly based on your opponent: do you think he has a better hand? Can you get a read off of him that indicates what cards he is holding? Before a race, we are often concerned with how we'll perform in comparison to others. Some of us try to beat our training partners. Others try for age group awards, while some are simply afraid of finishing dead last.

Obviously, the fear of losing is the most nerve-racking aspect of going all-in for professional card players. In no-limit poker, any given hand could result in sudden elimination. Similarly, with every race, runners risk failure or disappointment with a poor showing.

But just as there is no way to advance in the WSOP without going all-in, there is no better way to improve our performances than by putting everything on the line in a race. Any of us who are concerned with PRs, age group places, and comparative times from year to year need to go all-in on a regular basis – not just when we have the perfect hand.

Without the motivation of the next race looming over us, many of us would tend to ease up on our training, gradually losing our edge and our speed, the same way a pile of chips dwindles away one hand at a time if never risked.

Don't be afraid if racing gives you a major-league case of the jitters; that's the nature of competition. For gamblers, this is the "juice" that draws them to the table: the panicky tension, the drama of exhilarating highs and gut-wrenching lows based on the fall of the cards. Runners become hooked on racing in search of the same thrill - in fact, many coaches say that if you aren't terrified before a race, you aren't properly prepared for it.

So maybe runners and poker players have more in common than it first appears. Running also brings together people from disparate backgrounds.

Some of us are oddballs. And while there aren't quite as many fat guys in our group, we know plenty of runners with B.O. issues.

Runners often use the phrase "go all-out" to indicate giving their maximal effort in a race. Next time, try this: when you are lined up at the start line, envision yourself pushing a big stack of chips into the middle of the road, and commit yourself to going all-*in*.

The Marathon Bug

Let's say you've recently finished your first half-marathon, and your body is now reasonably well recovered. You feel a great sense of accomplishment from completing 13 miles, and you're feeling pretty darn good about your running life.

Maybe you look adoringly at your finisher's medal – and perhaps, every so often, you squint your left eye so that the word "half" is obscured, but "marathon" is still visible. Perhaps you find yourself wondering what it would take to get a medal that looked like that. Sometimes you talk yourself out of it, but the idea lingers, and preoccupies your thoughts with each passing day.

If this is you – congratulations! You've caught the marathon bug. Trust us, it probably won't go away. The only question now is, what should you do about it? How do you make the leap from 13.1 to 26.2?

The answer isn't as hard as you may think. In fact, you can probably have yourself ready in as little as five to six months.

Your first, most important step is to commit yourself NOW to reaching the goal. Go online and register for your goal race. Your motivation to train will be much greater after you've officially signed up. Where your money goes, your body is likely to follow.

Between now and race day, you'll gradually progress your training towards your marathon goal. At first, you don't have to change the number of days you run or the number of miles. The most important adjustment is to reserve one day per week for a marathon-specific training run.

For instance, during the next two months, do a long run of 10 or 12 miles every other weekend. On the opposite weekends, run three to five miles at a pace that's slightly faster than your target marathon pace. This isn't dramatically different than most half marathon training plans.

In your third month, your overall mileage will gradually build, as the length of your training runs increase. Long runs should be 14 to16 miles, and marathon pace workouts can be anywhere from 5 to 9 miles. Many runners will raise their mid-week mileage as well, but this depends on how your body responds to the longer weekend runs.

Once you reach your fourth month of training, long runs should be 14 to 16 miles in length, increasing to 16 to 18 miles in your fifth month. Your longest run should be three weeks before your goal race, and should be at least 22 miles.

Finally, don't hesitate to enlist some help. Find someone who runs marathons and pester them for advice. Use the Internet to find local running clubs, marathon training schedules, and online discussion groups.

Yes, the road is hard sometimes, but the rewards are worth it. If you thought the sense of accomplishment from running 13 miles was great – believe us, the pride of a marathon finish is exponentially more. And it's available to anyone who wants to make the leap.

If you're bitten by the marathon bug, be bold and scratch that itch. Chances are, it will never go away unless you do.

Through the Darkness

If you want to call yourself a marathon runner, one thing is certain: you're going to suffer for it.

Suffering just comes with the territory; it's part of the deal you sign up for when you choose to take on this particular event. And it doesn't matter how fast you are. To some degree or another, everybody – from the 5-minute milers to the back of the pack – goes through an extremely difficult stretch sometime during the marathon. If you are working hard and pushing your limits, you are bound to suffer.

At Big Sur, it's no surprise that most people run into trouble at the same part of the course – miles 21-23 through Carmel Highlands. This backbreaking stretch of steep rolling hills can completely demoralize the best of runners. It's the place where inner demons emerge, and our bodies cry out against the pain we inflict upon them to continue onward.

We've both had stretches through the Highlands when it feels like we can barely keep our legs moving. Sometimes, we create a visible target to reach before stopping for a walking break: just make it to the next cone, the next telephone pole, the base of the next hill. The marathon becomes a continuous series of 50-yard efforts, and it's all we can do to move from one to another.

Runners often call it "the wall," but it's also like entering a long, dark tunnel, where all of the bright, pleasant reasons you had for doing the marathon in the first place are blocked from your mind. Your focus becomes isolated on the multitude of negative signals your body is sending to the rational side of your brain. The only way through the darkness is to keep moving forward, and the only person who can get you there is you.

Again, this happens to virtually everyone. At Big Sur, the two of us have nearly killed ourselves on that road. We've run when our feet became torn up, our calves and quads were on fire, our stomachs were cramping, and it felt like our legs were made of lead. And to various degrees, on race day, three thousand other people were doing the exact same thing.

For some runners it's only a temporary slowdown; for others, it's a complete collapse. Yet somehow, we figure out a way to will our bodies onward, and eventually cross the finish line just like we knew we would all along.

Then a curious thing happens: in the aftermath, runners often talk about how disappointed they are to have succumbed to hopelessness and despair during those dark miles, even if they only faltered to a slight degree. But honestly, it's pointless to question it.

Because the real question should be, why *wouldn't* somebody's thoughts turn a bit negative under these circumstances? We can't imagine somebody going through similar physical conditions and being able to completely block out all of those psychological alarms.

It's almost like a chicken-and-egg scenario: do our thoughts turn bad because we are struggling physically, or do we struggle because we lose our mental focus?

The most sensible answer goes something like this: our physical training before the race prepares our bodies to carry us through the most difficult stretches of a marathon. The better our training is, the more efficiently (i.e., without losing too much time) we'll get through those dark miles. But that doesn't mean we won't encounter self-doubt or other mental anguish along the way. That particular obstacle is unavoidable, no matter how well-conditioned someone is.

But here's the funny part: going through that darkness is the part of the marathon that many runners appreciate the most.

Those of us who are hooked on this sport know that there is nothing more rewarding than working our bodies to the brink of failure and staring down our inner demons, then somehow pulling ourselves through to emerge triumphantly on the other side. Some finishers will tell you they don't even know how they get through those critical patches, yet they always find a way.

And every time we go through that fire, we gain a self-appreciation and self-respect that is (as MasterCard would say) truly priceless. What's more, we're thankful for the hardships that helped us earn such awareness, because they're not so easy to find in our everyday lives. Many people become addicted to the feeling, and start looking for another race to renew the fight all over again.

Those people are called marathoners.

Fountain of Youth

Any runner will tell you that age is just a number. Our local running club has about two dozen members who are in their seventies, many of whom can keep up with the youngsters. The younger runners don't see this as unusual at all; they know that age doesn't matter if someone can keep the pace.

Legendary Bay Area runner Jack Kirk ran the fabled Dipsea Race in Marin County a record 67 times, until he finally hung up his shoes and retired after completing the race a final time at age 95. The race starts with a climb up nearly 700 stairs – equivalent to the height of a fifty-story building – before rambling up and down mountainous trails and treacherous terrain for over 7 miles. Kirk once famously said, "You don't stop running because you get old. You get old because you stop running."

The Tarahumara Indians in the desolate Copper Canyons of the Mexican Sierra Madres are folk heroes of distance running. As Christopher McDougall describes in *Born to Run*, the Tarahumara reside in caves and adobe huts separated by great distances, and their only means of transportation is running on narrow footpaths up and down the steep canyons. Running is a key part of their culture, as kids play games where they run up to 100 miles at a time. Amazingly, their civilization knows no heart disease, cancer, stroke, diabetes, depression, or hypertension. Furthermore, many of their best runners are 50 to 60 years old.

The lesson from these stories is this: if you want to be healthy and productive in your golden years, one of the best things you can do for yourself is to get running. It's like sipping from a fountain of youth.

We've been very fortunate to train with a group of local septuagenarians who are a great example of this idea. They make running a daily activity. Instead of talking about ailments and medications, they talk about their next race or next vacation. Many of them are among the fastest seventy plus runners in the country – in fact, four of them have their sights set on a world record attempt for the 4 x 1500m relay in the near future. Another one runs up to 15 marathons per year, and some others have run every one of Big Sur's 24 previous marathons.

In addition to being great mentors to their younger training partners, all of these great older runners are perfect examples of how the benefits of running are available at any age. Even if you're in your fifties, sixties, or seventies, it's never too late to start! The fountain of youth is right before you; feel free to take a sip.

Bang the Doldrums

In the closing scene of *Finding Nemo*, the "tank gang" who resided in P. Sherman's dental office finally pulls off the escape they've dreamt about for years; after Dr. Sherman places them in plastic bags to change the tank water, they manage to roll their bags across the counter to an open window, freefall two stories to the ground below, and then roll across four lanes of traffic before plunging over the wharf and into the welcoming waters of Sydney Harbor.

After hitting the water, they all let out a celebratory cheer. But as they continue bobbing on the waves inside their plastic bags, they suddenly grow quiet and pensive. Just before the credits roll, Bloat the pufferfish (voiced by Brad Garrett) asks the question that is on all of their minds: "Now what?"

It's the same question many marathoners ask themselves after finishing a major race.

The tank gang had focused so much time and energy on accomplishing their task that they hadn't really considered what to do once they actually completed it. Similarly, many runners spend countless weeks and months of marathon training focused on achieving the goal – whether just finishing the race or setting a personal best - without giving much thought to what will happen after they cross the finish line.

It's simple human nature (and since the tank gang felt it, maybe fish nature as well) to feel directionless, or even to go through a mild funk after a big event. It becomes tough to find motivation for even the most basic workouts. Runners of all ages and abilities frequently struggle with finding inspiration to keep training, and before they know it, much of that fitness improvement is lost.

Luckily, there are many strategies that can kick-start your motivation for running, and the period when you have those post-race blues is the perfect time to try some of them out. Here are some suggestions:

Thank you sir, may I have another: This seems obvious, but the easiest way to stay focused on marathon training is to sign up for another event. In many areas of the country, there are races within a single day's drive almost every month of the year. Find a race online, pay your entry fee, and you'll be amazed at how quickly you feel compelled to start training again.

Change your game: If you've been focused on primarily one race distance, take on the challenge of an unfamiliar distance. Being a good 5K or 10K runner demands far different strengths and skills than marathoning does, and the variety in training is guaranteed to keep things interesting.

Conversely, if you're in a rut of doing the same 5K/10K races all the time, try stepping up in distance to the half or full marathon. If you've already got the speed, building endurance is usually a lot easier than you think.

Get spiked: Many running clubs host informal track meets, especially during the summer, and this is when many marathoners lace up their spikes to build their speed with short distance races.

How fast can you run a mile? How about a quarter mile? If you dedicate yourself to track workouts for a whole season, you might be amazed at how quickly you improve.

A fun bonus of track racing is that you can compare your times to local high school meets, to see how you stack up against the young guns. Just don't get too depressed if your best 800m time would only place you 6th in the "C" heat of the girls' JV meet. It's true what they say about aging, you know.

Play in the dirt: The popularity of trail running has become enormous in recent years, and the number of races all over the country has grown immensely as well. Trail races usually cater to beginners, with short race options and a laid-back attitude that doesn't emphasize speed – in fact, many trail races don't even give awards afterwards.

Get on the Internet and look for a local trail race in your area. The trail running experience is too good to miss; in fact; many runners enter their first trail race, and never return to roads again. Go and see what all the fuss is about.

Give it a tri: If you're really looking to supercharge your training, think about making the transition from runner to multisport athlete. Many runners already cross train with cycling and swimming – so it shouldn't be too much of a leap to consider entering a triathlon. If you've just finished a marathon, your fitness base is already good enough for most triathlons; just get some bike rides under your belt and find some pool access, and you'll be in business.

Wait it out: Sometimes lethargy is just your body's way of telling you that it needs a break, dummy. Runners, and marathoners in particular, often get so preoccupied with achieving certain goals that they ignore signs of cumulative fatigue until they become overwhelming.

If this is the case, just pamper yourself with a few weeks of lighter activity and extra sleep, and you may rediscover your motivation for getting back on the horse once your body has recharged its battery.

The tank gang from *Finding Nemo* eventually get out of the bags and enjoy their new lives in the ocean. Likewise, most runners usually snap out of their doldrums without doing anything unusually drastic. But if you're looking for a quicker solution, try one of our ideas above to keep training strong all throughout the year.

Running –Weather or Not!

Runners in our hometown on the Monterey Peninsula encounter very few days of unfavorable weather. However, we've both run in other areas of the country, on days of 100-degree heat or zero-degree cold, in thunderstorms or snow or sleet and hail. Sure, the conditions are potentially life threatening - but when you have to run, you have to run! There is virtually no excuse for avoiding an outdoor adventure by (gag) staying indoors on the treadmill, or even (heaven forbid) skipping your run altogether. The key is to have the right attitude and some basic preparation.

Part 1- Attitude

Remember when you were a kid, how much fun it was to play in the rain and stomp in the puddles? We never cared about being wet or getting our clothes muddy or feeling chilled to the bone when we finished. Running in foul weather is an easy way for grownups to recreate that childhood enthusiasm. Some of our most memorable running moments have occurred in adverse weather, to the point where we actually look forward to rain and wind sometimes when planning our runs.

A few years ago we both ran the Napa Valley Marathon in early March. The race started in light drizzle and about 40 degrees, and the weather turned progressively worse as the morning wore on. By mile 20 it was 32 degrees and hailing, and the monsoon-like headwinds gusted up to 40 miles per hour. The conditions were so bad that even the reliable aid station volunteers had abandoned their posts because of flying debris, yet most of the runners pressed onward. One of the most memorable moments occurred when a friend of ours showed classic determination as the storm howled and he approached the biggest hill of the course, looked up to the sky and yelled, "Is that ALL you've got?!!!"

Our friend's attitude is typical of many distance runners. He treated the horrible weather conditions as a challenge and with good humor. Runners are accustomed to overcoming obstacles. Heck, just completing a marathon in perfect weather is difficult. Doing so in bad conditions is a merely a further test of body, will, and spirit.

Our group of training partners has been running the same hilly 13-mile loop course virtually every Tuesday morning for the last 20 years. Mornings in the winter are frequently freezing and rainy but virtually everyone shows up. On the few occasions when there is actually snow accumulated – a somewhat rare sight in Monterey County - at the top of the biggest climb, we're more likely to break out into Christmas carols than gripe about the conditions. We're certainly not the most intrepid group of runners around, but we all understand that a run in bad conditions is a far better experience than skipping a workout on account of timidity.

Hugo Ferlito, the Big Sur International Marathon's Chairman of the Board, is famous for saying, "The course is flat and the weather is perfect!" Anyone who has run the extremely daunting Big Sur course knows differently, but most of us don't care. We understand that the headwinds are as much a part of the challenge as the rolling hills.

Some years the wind at Big Sur is just a pest, but other years it is diabolical. Most people think of Hurricane Point simply as a two-mile climb - but after all, there's a reason it is called *Hurricane* Point! We've seen runners blown over sideways and unable to stand upright at the top. Sometimes the wind carries sand and small pebbles that can leave your face raw and bruised for days afterward. People sometimes ask us if this really fun – and our answer is YES, if your attitude is right. It's all part of the challenge and mystique of the marathon.

Part 2 – Preparation

Nowadays, it is relatively easy to prepare for adverse conditions. Performance fabrics and specialized gear make it much easier to train in foul weather than ten years ago. Technical clothing is more expensive than the traditional cotton t-shirts and sweats we grew up with, but it is far more effective at keeping you dry and warm during your run.

In cold weather, many novice runners make the mistake of wearing too much clothing. Even in frigid weather, after about 10 minutes of running you can feel fairly comfortable with just two top layers – such as a long sleeve shirt and a weatherproof jacket - with pants, gloves, and a stocking hat as accessories. Dressing in light layers allows for more effective temperature regulation as your body warms up.

Rain is a bit trickier, as it is extremely hard to stay dry even on drizzly days. Rain-resistant jackets often become too warm once your body heats up, so some people like to wear a lightweight technical top layer, and just be prepared to get wet. Others like the old-school approach of wearing a poncho, or even a standard plastic garbage bag with holes cut out for your head and arms to keep your trunk dry and warm while allowing your arms and legs to get soaked.

Our theory is that you're going to sweat from the inside anyway, so just pick the clothing ensemble you prefer and brace yourself for the initial discomfort of the first mile. Once you've run for a short time, the conditions start to feel much more comfortable, and in our opinion, they even become quite enjoyable.

No matter what time of year you are training, the weather could turn nasty, so you had better be prepared for it. The next time conditions are bad, don't let them stop you - just gear up, and get out there and enjoy your run! Don't forget to stomp in the puddles.

ROADSIDE PHILOSOPHY

"When runners get injured, we feel like the sky is falling. We get depressed and feel inadequate and our problems take on irrational dimensions. Yet those are precisely the times we should remember just how lucky we are."

"For certain, the wheel in the sky will keep on turning, and one of these days we won't be out there for a weekly loop. But until then, we'll continue to mark the passing of the years and the changes they bring – or don't bring – one week at a time on Tuesday mornings."

Find Happiness

Before a big race, it's always interesting to hear what people have to say.

Sometimes when we're counting down the days to a marathon or long trail race, we receive e-mails and texts from friends wishing us success in the upcoming event. Our running friends recognize how many months are spent in preparation beforehand, and they can all sympathize with our pre race jitters and anticipation.

Most friends say things like "good luck," "run fast," or the ever-popular "may the wind be at your back." Others try to build your confidence by saying "You've done all the training, now enjoy the race," or "You're strong and ready – go do it!"

Fortunately, for obvious reasons, runners never abide by the traditional good luck message used by the theatre community: "Break a leg!"

Some running veterans offer messages that are wise, simple, and can be used as a mantra during the race: "patience"; "determination"; "strong and smooth"; "run smart." Two Monterey County Olympians, Alvin and Calvin Harrison, used to instruct each other to "run to your destiny" before each race.

Having run many races over the years, we thought we had received every possible well-wishing message – but our friend Jon surprised us recently. Before an important marathon, Mike had been complaining about various aches and pains; maybe he was looking for sympathy, or perhaps subconsciously making early excuses for a less than perfect run.

Jon sent him an e-mail simply saying, "Find happiness."

Return message from Mike: "Very Zen … you must be joking!"

Jon's reply: "I'm not joking, Grasshopper."

The unspoken implication is that virtually every marathoner has aches and pains before a big event, and every race is a challenge the runner voluntarily decides to enter. At any time before the starting gun goes off, it's possible to simply decide not to run – however, even with lowered expectations, the satisfaction of finishing the marathon is always a great thrill.

In light of this, it's quite helpful to consider your reasons for racing in the first place. Is it a method for you to find happiness? And if the endeavor isn't ultimately enjoyable for you, then why do it? Mike's mantra for that marathon became, "Don't worry, be happy," which helped carry him all the way through the race. It's amazing how a focused mind can mask all kinds of physical aches and pains.

As you make your training plans, take a few minutes to contemplate why you run. Resolve to find joy in your life and in your running. Be thankful for how lucky you are for your health and ability to exercise.

Runners usually set goals that involve checking various races off our to-do list or improving our personal best times – but along with those things, be sure to celebrate your running and fitness throughout the year. Savor the miles spent with friends, the beautiful places you encounter, and the freedom to do the activities you enjoy. Play a bit more, and be serious a little less.

Running's "first philosopher," George Sheehan, once said, "Every mile I run is my first. Every hour on the roads is a new beginning. Every day I put on my running clothes, I am born again. Seeing things as if for the first time, seeing the familiar as unfamiliar, the common as uncommon."

Go see those things for yourself. Run for the joy of it. And find happiness.

Best Running Lessons

Often the best running lessons you learn are also your best life lessons – and one of the great benefits of running is that every time you step out the door you may learn something valuable. Strangely, my best running lesson happened before I (Mike) was a runner, and to this day I'm still learning from it.

My best friend growing up in San Jose and in college at Berkeley was Paul. Paul had polio when he was a kid but recovered and became a great athlete. He had tremendous eye-hand coordination and excelled in all aspects of sport thanks to that skill. He would beat me and everyone else like a drum, either shooting hoops, playing golf, pitching and hitting the baseball, as quarterback on the football field, or goofing around at ping pong.

But Paul wasn't that big and was fairly overweight. His leg speed was legendary but for the wrong reasons. All the proper nicknames applied: molasses, ice flow, continental drift. He was slow with a capital S, L, O, and W.

Paul headed off to Santa Barbara for his last few years of college and came back a different person. He grew several inches and started running before running was cool. When I saw him, after a year break, he was a different person; slim, tan, and more confident. When he challenged me to a running race I thought he was joking.

A running race? Certainly I could never lose to "molasses" Paul. But why not do it? He wanted to race two miles on the track the next day and I started my bidding at 200 yards in two weeks. This race could very well be won or lost in the negotiation stages. We decided it would be fun to settle on the classic mile distance. No spectators, either – just mano a mano. San Jose City College track in a week.

I trained a bit over the next week, but really knew very little about running. Race day was very warm and I decided the best strategy was to just stay at whatever pace Paul was running and then outkick him with a hundred yards to go. I had no doubt I would win. Paul was S. L. O. W.

The first lap was pretty tactical and I was very comfortable running alongside him. There was a lot of trash talk and he actually seemed to be laughing at me and smirking. He picked up the pace gradually on laps 2 and 3 and seemed very comfortable as I was gasping for breath and struggling by the end of lap 3. On the last lap he forged ahead about 10 yards, then 20, then more, and I could visualize myself defeated and demoralized. Losing to Paul would be a lifetime setback.

But just like in the movies, with my heart pounding, legs and arms like lead, I willed myself closer. My body said NO with every step, and then started yelling "Hell NO!" but my mind was stronger. It was a complete surprise and I put on a finishing kick and passed him with about 30 yards to go.

I had learned huge lessons that day. The human body can do miraculous things if you let it. Strength of will can carry you to success. More importantly, I should have prepared more. There is great personal satisfaction in striving to be your best.

Now, forty some odd years later, I am still learning from that lesson and from Paul. He is now thought to have post-polio syndrome; a disease where the ravages of polio return later in life. Muscle weakness, trouble walking, labored breathing, nerve damage, all return. My father was also a polio victim as a child and had the same debilitating disease later in life. It's vastly unfair; especially so because they were both athletes.

While Paul now has trouble breathing and walks using a walker, I can run marathons. While Paul takes tons of prescribed medications, I choose to take vitamins. While every effort is a struggle for Paul, I find things easy. While he is depressed and pessimistic, I am upbeat and optimistic. Certainly in his condition I would be depressed and pessimistic as well. Probably more than he is.

Do I feel guilty for being healthy? Yes I do. Am I powerless to help? Yes again. Do I feel guilty that I can't help? Absolutely! Do I feel lucky to be healthy and in control of this luck? Unfortunately, I don't. It seems to be the luck of the draw; random in every way.

Looking back on this seemingly unimportant mile race at San Jose City College 40 years ago, I now realize the biggest lesson was that I was in a situation where I ultimately controlled the outcome. My own will pulled me through. Also I realize that if Paul had been faster or better trained, I could have tried my best and still finished second, but I still would have known inside that I did my best. No guilt. No random acts. The win wasn't the lesson, it was the total effort. It was about control.

Everytime I run now I feel totally in control and healthy. No guilt. Life is fair.

It's when I stop that I have my doubts.

Dear Santa

Dear Santa,

We hope this letter finds you well, and that your final preparations for Christmas Eve are going smoothly.

Hopefully you remember us – we're the running columnists from Monterey County who wrote to you last year with a wish list of things that could make us better runners. We've had a pretty good year, Santa – but we've also seen a lot of things that make us sad about our favorite sport, and we were hoping that you could possibly help us again this year. Incidentally, many other sports face the same problems that running does, so if you can fix these things, you'd have the admiration of millions of sports fans around the world. (Not that you don't have it already).

We believe in you, Santa, and we want to believe in our sport also. Unfortunately, this seems harder to do with each passing year. In light of this, would the following things be too much to ask?

The excitement of true fans: We used to love watching national collegiate or professional championship events, world championships and Olympics – but in recent years, we've grown pretty jaded. We don't know whether to appreciate the feats we witness on the TV screen anymore. We used to watch with a sense of awe and wonder – but now we just wonder. Maybe it's because we're lacking …

Faith in hard work: When we watched sports as kids, there was always an underlying premise that success was available to anyone with God-given talent and the willingness to work hard toward his or her goals. Lately, as top-level athletes in every sport are getting busted for various forms of cheating, it seems like skills and dedication are only part of the equation. It also makes us lose our …

Belief in records: Here's how bad things have become: whenever we see a record get broken, or hear of a performance for the ages by a star athlete, our first reaction isn't to say, "Wow, I'm watching history!" but to ask, "I wonder what that guy's using." This happens with alarming frequency in nearly every sport. Who was the last truly clean 100-meter dash world record holder, Tour de France champion, or baseball home run king? Nobody knows for certain – which makes every current and future record a cause for skepticism rather than celebration.

You know what might help, Santa? Maybe if we could get some …

Professional athletes giving back to the fans: Wouldn't it be refreshing if some of our highest-paid superstars started saying, "You know, I could live quite comfortably on eight million a year instead of eighteen million; why not use the extra ten million to get free game tickets for kids, or to lower everyone's cost by $5.00 a ticket."

And all this new altruism just might be contagious and result in…

Honesty from cheaters: Just once – just one time – this year, we'd like to hear someone who tests positive for performance enhancing drugs come out and say, "You know what? You caught me. I was cheating, and I was wrong to do it. I did it because I have to compete against a lot of other guys I know who are also cheating – and here are their names. I'm sorry, I shouldn't have done it, and I'll accept whatever punishment you decide is fair." Could you imagine how refreshing that would be? It would be one small step towards restoring the notion of …

Athletes as role models: We're thinking of runners in particular here. Remember a long time ago, when the most famous athletes in the world were Roger Bannister or Jim Ryun or Bill Rodgers? Nowadays, most people would have trouble naming an Olympic gold medalist in any distance event over the past 20 years. Running has completely fallen off the radar. But there are several young American runners today with world-class talent. Maybe if they become more popular, we might also see …

Respect for runners: It seems like there's always been this notion that distance runners are the misfits of the athletic world, since they don't often participate in more glamorous sports like football or basketball.

But take it from us, Santa: distance running is hard work. Cross-country is a brutal sport – and those skinny runners are just as intense and competitive as any 220-pound linebacker. They push themselves beyond boundaries of pain that most other athletes dare not approach, and they do it almost anonymously. We'd just like more people to understand that.

Well, Santa, you've got your work cut out for you. Sorry to make this list so challenging, but we figured that we'd rather have meaningful change rather than toys and gadgets that we don't really need anyway. We know we won't get everything we ask for, but anything you can do to make the world a better place for runners would be greatly appreciated.

Thanks for your time, Santa. Have a safe flight on Christmas Eve!

Sincerely,

Mike and Donald

Monterey County, CA

Avoiding Bad Juju

Marathon racing is complicated business. You have to start conservatively, check your split times obsessively, pace yourself well through the early miles, manage your fluid and caloric intake, and deal with the discomfort and despair of running through "the wall." The last thing you want to do is make your race more troublesome by inviting bad juju.

Juju is a term adopted from African culture, with various meanings that are somewhat related to superstition. It can be a charm or object with magical powers, or any ritual act that influences the forces of nature for better or worse.

As it relates to running, juju is a specific behavior that really shouldn't have any affect on race performance, but inevitably does. However, it's important to point out that acts which directly affect physical performance, such as inadequate training, improper race preparation or foolish strategy, do not count. For example, wearing a new pair of shoes on race day or eating something unfamiliar before the race isn't bad juju - it's just stupidity.

But juju is nothing to be taken lightly; mess around with it too much, and you're just inviting disaster. Experienced marathon runners are careful to avoid bad juju before and during their event –and here are a few of the most common examples:

Rule #1: Predicting your own race time is bad juju. This is the "pride goeth before the fall" postulate of juju. On race day, there are too many variables that can conspire against you, to assume that they will all come down in your favor. Nevertheless, runners of all speeds frequently break this rule. As soon as you state "I'll probably run in *x* amount of time," you are almost guaranteeing yourself a finish time that is much slower.

Try this experiment: ask a veteran marathoner how fast they are going to run an upcoming race. If they know anything about juju, they will hem and haw and be as evasive as a crooked politician whenever you try to pin them down to a specific answer. To avoid bad juju, never forecast a specific time. It's much safer to say, "I'm hoping to run *x* time," or "My goal is to run it in *x* time"; statements that don't tempt fate nearly as much as a declared specific prediction.

Rule #2: Wearing the shirt of the exact race you are running is bad juju. This falls under the "don't count your chickens before they hatch" category of juju. It's never acceptable to wear the t-shirt for the race until after you have actually completed it. Just because you show up at the marathon expo and pick up your packet doesn't guarantee that you'll finish the race the next morning. Unforeseen injuries, stomach cramps, blisters, or a myriad of other problems can quickly lead to a DNF - and when that happens, you'll be stuck there at the side of the road, advertising the event that just kicked your butt.

It would be like the losing team deciding to go ahead and wear those "Super Bowl Champs" hats that are printed in advance for each team, but only given to the winners. How ridiculous would that look? That's the risk you run by wearing the race shirt during the event. (By the way, what happens to all of those unusable hats and t-shirts? Hopefully they're sent to impoverished villages somewhere that don't have TV or Internet access. There must be a whole society in some remote corner of the world that thinks the Buffalo Bills won four Super Bowls).

Rule #3: Wearing the shirt from one race while racing in another is bad juju. The worst mistake a runner can make is underestimating or disrespecting any given course. In order to race well, you have to focus all of your energy on the challenge at hand, and not look ahead to the next race, or dwell excessively on a past event. Wearing the shirt from another marathon demonstrates conflicting interests and loyalties. It's the equivalent of going out to a special dinner with your girlfriend, while wearing a sweater that was an anniversary gift from a previous lover, and having your current girlfriend recognize it. This is the "how can you be committed to me when you're thinking of another girl?" tenet of juju.

The only exception to this rule that we may consider is if the race distance of the shirt you are wearing is longer than the distance you are currently racing. Some people do this to psych themselves up during rough stretches, saying, "If I finished that race, I can finish this one." However, this is a somewhat unreliable crutch, as we've passed many people wearing Ironman singlets or Western States Endurance Run shirts who looked desperately exhausted while racing at Big Sur.

Rule #4: Telling your finish line posse that you'll be done at a certain time is bad juju. This is a more severe variant of Rule #1. It could be called contagious juju because it affects not just you, but everyone who is awaiting your arrival at the finish line as well. Imagine the worry and embarrassment inflicted on your spouse and friends when they are looking for you, but you are nowhere to be found. Progressively bad thoughts cross their minds for every minute you are delayed beyond your predicted arrival time. When you finally arrive, instead of finding people who are sympathetic to your bad day, you'll be facing an angry or stressed-out mob. Instead of being a hero, you are merely late and a bearer of bad juju. To avoid this plight, give your loved ones an approximate window of arrival times.

These are the most obvious cases of bad juju in action, but we're really just scratching the surface with these examples. We recognize that there's no rational explanation for these phenomena, but we've had enough experiences and observations to firmly believe in the power of juju. Running a marathon is hard enough on its own – so follow our advice, respect the juju, and don't ruin all of your hard training with foolhardy behaviors that can tip the scales of karma against you.

Time Passages

The rock band Journey once sang, "The wheel in the sky keeps on turning/ I don't know where I'll be tomorrow." And while that may be true, the two of us know one thing for certain: if that wheel rises on a Tuesday, we'll be meeting at 5:25 AM for our training group's regularly scheduled 13-mile run on the outskirts of Salinas.

"The Loop" is a signature route for our running group, and it's an intimidating run even for the best local runners. It's a hilly, challenging route, and there's no mercy shown for stragglers. If you show up one minute late, you have to catch up. If you're having an off day, you'll get dropped by the start of the first climb. Despite all this, there is a core group that has been doing the loop consistently for more than two decades. Mike joined the group a few years after its inception, and has been one of its mainstays for over 16 years now.

But the wheel in the sky turns differently for everyone, so the surrounding cast of characters who accompany Mike has changed in that period of time. However, the following excerpts from Mike's training logs illustrate that while some things change, others remain more constant.

* * *

Last Tuesday in November 1989: There are five of us running the loop this morning.

We're all 42 or 43 except Doug, who is 37 and the fastest of the group. We only keep up with him because he is polite, and because he sometimes stops in the bushes for a "sabbatical" and then catches up later.

Don drops behind on the uphills but catches up on the downs. Jim E. falls behind on the downhills but presses the pace on the ups and catches up. I run consistently with Marc, who grunts and groans while talking constantly.

We talk about our kids and work and Monday Night Football. We tell a lot of jokes. We discuss our last races and upcoming ones. We solve some of the world's problems. Our loop time of 1:31:45 feels pretty easy, and is about the average time for 1989. Everyone piles into their cars and heads off to work.

* * *

Last Tuesday in November 1999: There are five of us running the loop this morning.

I'm 52. Jefferson is 45. Donald is the youngest at 29. Jim S. and Keith are 35. Jim is the fastest of the group and we only keep up with him because he is polite, and because he sometimes stops in the bushes for a sabbatical before catching up later.

Jefferson drops behind on the uphills but catches up on the downs. Donald falls behind on the downhills but presses the pace on the ups to catch us. I run consistently with Keith, who grunts and groans when he's not talking dirty.

We talk about our kids and work and Monday Night Football. We tell jokes that most of us have heard before. We discuss our last races and upcoming ones. We solve most of the world's problems. Our loop time of 1:34:28 is about average for 1999, and left me pretty tired but Donald seemed refreshed. It was a pretty easy run for Jim and Keith, who continue running a few more miles to warm down while the rest of us head off to work.

* * *

Last Tuesday in November 2005: There are eleven of us running the loop this morning. I'm now 58 and retired, but I like to get up early to meet the group anyway. We run together for the first mile or so then quickly break up into two groups of five.

The faster pack has Donald who is 35. Dave, Andrew, Keith and Mark are 41. Ben is 31. Dave is the fastest of the group, and the others keep up with him only because he is polite, and occasionally stops in the bushes for a sabbatical before catching up later.

Andrew and Dave go off the front during the final miles. Ben drops behind on the uphills but catches up on the downs. Mark falls behind on the downhills but presses the pace on the ups and catches up. Donald runs consistently with Keith, who grunts and groans and still talks dirty. The group picks up the pace in the final miles for loop times between 1:29 and 1:31, which is pretty comfortable for the faster runners.

I run with the slower pack that includes my son Bryan who is 30. Carmella is 35. Cobi is the youngster at 28. Steve is 51. Cobi drops behind on the uphills but catches up on the downs. Bryan falls behind on the downhills but presses the pace on the ups and catches up. Carmella and Steve and I run together. The pace makes me grunt and groan occasionally, but at least I don't talk dirty.

Both groups talk about kids and work and Monday Night Football. I talk about my grandkids. We talk about our last races and upcoming ones. We tell a few jokes – all of which we've heard before – and solve all of the world's problems. My group runs 1:38:11, which is a struggle for me in the last few miles.

Everyone goes to work, but I go home and sit down to read a book after breakfast, and then fall asleep in the chair.

* * *

Undoubtedly, the wheel in the sky will keep on turning, and one of these Tuesdays mornings we won't be out there for the weekly loop. But until then, we'll continue to mark the passing of the years and the changes they bring – or don't bring – one week at a time on Tuesday mornings.

Remembrance of a Runner

A recent obituary in the Herald honored a 55-year-old woman named Belinda, whose "natural friendliness, kindness, generosity, and good cheer made her many friends." It mentioned that her passions in life included her cats, arts and crafts, and the company of friends.

One other note caught our attention; it stated that Belinda "was especially proud of completing the Big Sur International Marathon."

Truth be told, it's not the first time we've noticed a line like that in the obituaries – but for some reason, this one made us reflect a bit on life experiences we share.

What defines you? What accomplishment are you most proud of? How do others think of you? When people describe you to others, what will they say?

On the rare occasions that we get recognized around town from our smiling pictures above this column – believe us, it doesn't happen that often - it's usually followed by the comment, "Oh…you're that runner dude." Or sometimes, more simply, "You're the runner."

Even at work or in social situations, friends and acquaintances define us most easily as "the runner." We're not always sure how to take this, seeing as how we both have advanced educational degrees, professional careers, loving families, and are active in our religious communities, among other activities we enjoy. But apparently we're not as noteworthy at anything else as we are at running.

It's also curious to note that earlier in life, Donald was known as "the rower", and Mike as "the golfer." Most of our friends from those times were defined the same way. The sport you practice or activity you enjoy are often the most visible, and therefore the most easily identifiable aspects of how other people see us.

All this brings us back to the obituaries, which are always an interesting place to see how people are defined by others. Loved ones who write them offer their personal views of the departed's accomplishments, priorities, and joys in life. Appropriately, the person's family role is mentioned first: loving husband; father of three; doting grandparent. An occupation is frequently listed soon thereafter. But inevitably, the person's activities and hobbies are described in some detail. And every now and then, you'll see a mention of our local marathon.

We've written countless times about how training for and completing a marathon can be a life-changing experience. It's an accomplishment that anyone should be proud of, and a milestone that outside observers recognize as significant. For most people, running 26.2 miles means more than just placing one foot in front of the other – it's a life-defining exercise that reveals and defines the person we are for all the world to see.

Belinda's obituary described how she "carried the burdens of developmental disabilities with great dignity, perseverance, and courage and would not let her challenges defeat her." She sounds like someone we're proud to call a fellow marathoner – and she's also a great example of what any of us can become.

The benefits and opportunities of running are available to anyone. You don't have to be born a natural athlete, and you don't have to be uniquely gifted. A life-shaping experience is there for the taking, waiting right outside your door. Maybe one of these years, you'll even finish a marathon – and if you do, it's an honor you can carry forever.

And if someone happens to refer to you one day as "the runner", don't take it the wrong way – just smile and consider it a compliment.

World's Hardest Course

There is a lot of debate in the running community about the world's most challenging foot race – and today, we're going to propose an unconventional entry to the discussion.

Sure, the very hilly Big Sur Marathon is tough – but it doesn't even make the "A" list of toughest running events. Ultramarathons such as the Western States Endurance Run command a lot of respect, but that particular course is considered a relatively "easy" 100-miler by some ultra runners, especially compared to ultras in the mountains of Colorado or Utah.

There's a marathon at Mount Everest and one in Antarctica. There's a 135-mile race through Death Valley, and a multi-day race where runners cross the Sahara Desert. It seems there's no limit to the insane conditions runners will subject themselves to.

Considering that partial list of nominees, our submission for the hardest running event on Earth will undoubtedly surprise you. From Mike's experience, the hardest running course known to man could be (drumroll, please) The 4-Year-Old Run.

This is the name Mike uses for a typical run with his two 4-year-old grandsons. Jeremy lives in Oakland and Devon in Sacramento – and although the houses are different, the running events are remarkably similar.

It always starts the same way: "Come on Grandpa, let's go for a run!" And the little ones immediately take off running from the living room as fast as their little legs can go. Mike gives chase, and the race of survival is on.

"You have to jump over Elmo!" they say, as well as about 10 other toys randomly assorted around the carpet. Then it's a few steps on and over the ottoman and into the dining room.

"You have to spin three times!" is usually the next comment. With spinning out of the way they crawl under the dining room table and chairs, waiting impatiently for Mike's bigger body to squeeze underneath the chairs. Then for good measure, it's around the table 5 times, until Mike is wishing he was running up Hurricane Point or across the Sahara Desert instead. "Come on Grandpa!"

Exiting the dining room, another complicating factor is added. The family dog is now yapping joyously and getting tangled in Mike's feet as he continues trying to catch the 4-year-olds.

Then it's on to the kitchen segment of the run. "You have to slide like this," they say, with hands out for balance, and socks sliding on the kitchen floor. Hips become sore from banging on the cabinets as Mike slides back and forth across the kitchen several times.

Then it's back to the living room and over the toys to complete the circuit. But wait! There's more torture coming. "You have to do this Grandpa." Mike watches incredulously as they jump as high as they can in the air, throw both feet straight out in front of them, and land flat on their little butts.

"I can't do THAT," he pleads.

"You HAVE to do that," they repeat. So Mike does that as best he can without causing severe butt and spine damage.

"No, you didn't do it right."

Mike tries to do THAT several more times until he's given a reluctant passing mark, given more out of the kids' boredom than respecting the quality of the jump. As he lies in pain on the floor, he knows from experience what is invariably coming next.

"AGAIN!" The dreaded "again" means that another circuit is starting with another furious sprint and jump over Elmo. The "agains" can be infinite and don't stop until Mike is mercifully saved by his laughing wife, saying "Let Grandpa rest. He seems really tired."

Mike rests on the floor exhausted, realizing that it's a blessing that the running life keeps him in shape to do the 4-Year-Old Run. It may be one of the most difficult events around, but he wouldn't have it any other way.

The Mountain of Erised

Tomorrow I (Donald) am flying to Colorado to run the Pikes Peak Marathon: a brutal 26.4-mile trail race up to the mountain's 14,110' summit and back down again. The race bills itself as "America's Ultimate Challenge," and many runners have suffered altitude sickness, dehydration, and heat stroke from the environment and climate, as well as scrapes, bruises, ankle sprains and broken bones from the sometimes-treacherous footing. Honestly, I can't wait – just typing these things makes me giddy.

Most runners probably understand the attraction, but occasionally my non-running acquaintances ask the simple question: why do you do it? Since we're in the midst of another summer of *Harry Potter* mania, I often find myself pulling an illustration from the book in reply.

The best way for me to explain it is that Pikes Peak is similar to the Mirror of Erised from the book series. In *Harry Potter and the Sorcerer's Stone*, Harry discovers the mirror stashed away in a dark, abandoned storage area at the Hogwarts School of Witchcraft and Wizardry. An inscription in mirror writing (of course) above it reads *Erised stra ehru oyt ube cafru oyt on wohsi* (read backwards: "I show not your face, but your heart's desire").

The mirror is a plot device to reveal the character of anyone who gazes upon it, rather than reflecting what's externally visible. Harry, who has never known his true family, sees his parents and extended family standing beside him in the mirror. His friend Ron, who is constantly overshadowed by several older siblings, sees himself achieving individual recognition for his accomplishments.

However, the mirror's revelations can also be dangerous. As Headmaster Dumbledore explains, "Men have wasted away before it, entranced by what they have seen, or been driven mad, not knowing if what it shows is real or even possible."

In the book's final chapter, the mirror is realized to be the hiding place of the Sorcerer's Stone, a magical creation that gives everlasting life to its keeper. Harry obtains the stone while in the clutches of the evil wizard Voldemort; staring at the mirror, Harry watches his reflection hold up the stone, then drop it into his pocket. He immediately reaches inside his pocket to feel the real stone in his grasp, and successfully manages to keep it away from Voldemort until it can be destroyed.

Pikes Peak in Colorado has the same effect on me as the mirror does for students at Hogwarts. I have a postcard of the peak taped on the wall just above my computer screen at work. When my mind wanders, I find myself staring at the mountain and considering what is reflected back at me. What I usually see in the mountain is everything my heart desires.

Before I learned about this race, I had never climbed a mountain before. I had never spent time at high altitude. I had never run for more than five hours (the average men's finishing time at this marathon is over seven hours). And yet, these were all abilities that I believed I had within me. I dearly wanted to experience them, and nearly every day during my training I envisioned myself running on the high mountain.

The race requires diligent preparation. My flatlander training consists of weekly 3-hour treadmill runs at 15% grade, and 4-to-5-hour runs up and down the canyons of my hometown of Carmel Valley, along with as much mileage as I can tolerate on the "easier" days. These efforts are physically demanding, but over the course of several weeks they also forge psychological strengths such as discipline, courage, and perseverance – all of which will be called upon on race day.

A training regimen like this can be dangerous in a somewhat insidious manner, as it potentially consumes other aspects of your life. Just as some men waste away staring endlessly at the Mirror of Erised, it's easy to let basic things like family time, home repairs, and social obligations (to say nothing of work productivity) fall by the wayside while spending an entire summer preparing to take on the mountain. Sometimes it almost requires a hand on the back of my shirt to yank my concentration back to my daily routine.

When I first started training for Pikes Peak, a small voice in my head asked if the qualities I saw in the mountain – and by reflection, in myself – were truly there, or whether they were even possible to attain. I was searching for something within myself, but had to travel to a faraway place for the answers. Would I find the things I was looking for? Would I even make it to the top to find out?

The attributes that enable you to reach the top of Pikes Peak sometimes aren't apparent until race day, when you finally stand upon the summit and take in how far – literally and figuratively – you have come, and how high you have climbed. You suddenly see all those positive things in yourself, as crystal clear as looking at your reflection in a mirror.

At that moment, in that place, it's like all of your toil and determination and resiliency converge upon you like a gift that's dropped into your pocket. If you're smart, you grasp those feelings like they're a Sorcerer's Stone, and carry them with you as far as possible on your trip down the mountain and back into your everyday life.

Unfortunately, the feeling doesn't last nearly as long as you would like it to, and at some point you'll inevitably want to chase it again. You encounter the same obstacles each time around. Even having completed the race before, those questions I had about myself the first time are present again this year. I stare at my Pikes Peak postcard every day, hoping the answers are still waiting for me at the summit.

That's why the Pikes Peak Marathon calls me back: it's my Mountain of Erised. It reveals the person I am capable of being. It displays parts of my character that aren't always apparent in my day to day life. And whenever I look at the mountain, it reflects my heart's desire to see and feel those things all over again.

THE STARTING LINE

"One of the most effective ways to fitness and health is to start running. It can be done anywhere, by nearly everybody, with minimal equipment needs. Besides being fun, it is the most efficient brand of exercise imaginable, and the benefits to your body are immeasurable."

"How would you like people to describe you as you grow older; as a couch potato or an athlete? Do you want to be a role model to those who follow you, or an example of behaviors to avoid? Those types of decision should be easy ones at any age."

Why and How

If you are one of the countless Americans who have decided to lose weight and exercise more often, congratulations – and good luck. It can be a difficult task. Our best advice is to simplify your exercise program to ensure success.

One of the most effective ways to fitness and health is to start running. It can be done anywhere, by nearly everybody, with minimal equipment needs. Besides being fun, it is the most efficient brand of exercise imaginable, and the benefits to your body are immeasurable. For example:

General Health: Running lowers your risk of heart disease and cancer, reduces blood pressure and stress levels, and improves your bone density. Among runners, the risk of nearly every significant cardiovascular disease is substantially reduced. Running has also been shown to improve the mental acuity of older runners, so it can actually make you smarter! Numerous medical studies have demonstrated the benefits of a regular running program.

Appearance: Running is the fastest way to lower your overall weight and improve your long-term weight management. Gradually, you'll notice a decreased waist size or dress size, along with enhanced muscle tone. Running can even improve your skin tone and hair thickness.

Social benefits: Running typically makes you feel better about yourself, and improves the way you interact with others. Running with a group is a great way to increase your social interaction and develop new friendships.

Outdoor experience: Yes, you can run indoors if you like, but most runners become hooked on the natural beauty of our surroundings. You can explore your neighborhood, tour your local parks, wander through forests, cruise along the beach, or enjoy scenic vistas from hilltop trails.

On the trails, you'll encounter some occasional wildlife, and on the roads, you'll see some colorful characters from time to time. There's no limit to the surroundings you might encounter.

Athletic outlet: Many runners channel their competitive natures through races. When you race, you see exactly where you stand in comparison to runners of similar age and gender. Most runners also keep track of their times and try to improve from one year to the next.

* * *

So, that's the WHY of getting started. Here's the HOW:

As a new runner, the most fundamental concerns are buying a pair of shoes and finding a place to run.

Obviously, the most crucial piece of equipment is a pair of shoes. Selecting the proper running shoes helps you run more comfortably, and decreases your chance of developing injuries. Also, shoe technology has become very sport-specific, so that perfect pair you use for tennis or aerobics won't do you much good for running.

The best pair of shoes to buy varies with each individual, based on factors that you may never have thought of: Do you pronate? Are your arches high or low? Are you a heel striker? What surfaces will you run on? The seemingly simple task of selecting a pair of shoes quickly becomes complicated. That's why you should go to a specialty running store where experts can address all of these issues and more (such as proper running clothing).

Go to a local running store and tell them you are a beginner looking for the right shoes, and they'll assist with everything you need. You can try on different brands and styles of shoes, and go for a short run outside the store in each pair.

Anticipate paying between $70 and $95 for a good, basic pair. Since this is the most important investment in your development as a runner, it's usually money well spent. However, don't feel compelled to buy the most expensive shoes, either- anything over $100 is too much for a first-time runner.

Walk around in your new shoes for a while to break them in – but after your first run, use your running shoes *only* for running. They will last longer and support you better this way.

Once you're ready to start running, there are plenty of places to begin.

If you're uncertain about your ability to run for short distances, start outside your own home, or at a local track. At the track, alternate one lap or even one-half lap of running with an equal amount of walking. On the road, alternate a few minutes of running with time spent walking. Gradually increase the running, and decrease or eliminate the walking intervals.

Start comfortably and don't overdo it initially. Be patient and you will gradually improve over time. Don't expect a "runner's high" on your first day, but allow yourself several weeks or more to develop a comfort zone.

For those who feel ready to run more than a few miles, the best way to get acquainted with the sport is to run with a group. Don't feel intimidated because you are a beginner; most runners are extremely welcoming to anyone who wants to join in. Runners love to answer questions and give advice to newcomers. No matter what speed you run, there will probably be somebody else who keeps a similar pace and can give you details of the group's schedule and running routes. Be forewarned – runners tend to be early risers and they are also somewhat compulsive. Runs will typically start promptly at the indicated times, so arrive a bit early to meet the other runners.

Once you meet other runners, you have a whole network of people who can assist you in meeting your long-term fitness goals. Have fun getting started, and begin enjoying the benefits of your new, healthier lifestyle!

Getting Started

Regular aerobic exercise is one of the best things you can ever do for yourself. It doesn't matter if you're a walker, jogger, in-line skater, marathon runner, or swimmer. We wouldn't even mind if you're a cyclist. The point is to pick an activity, and get out there and do it!

Of course, the two of us are partial to running, and we're determined to find ways to get new people joining us. That's why we describe the joy that running provides, and the excitement we feel when racing. We talk about the camaraderie we find from our fellow runners, and how being runners influences the way we see the world.

We recognize that starting a new running program can be tough, but don't be intimidated by the notion of becoming a runner. Everybody has to start somewhere. The most important thing is to be determined. Make up your mind that you will succeed, and then go about the process of improvement.

Here are some tips to help you get started:

Schedule your workout time. If it's difficult to find time for running, make an appointment with yourself just as you would an important meeting at work. The specific time of day doesn't matter. Try for three "appointments" per week. For newcomers, anything between 5 and 30 minutes of running is plenty.

Don't think of it as a "program" or "project." Exercise should just be something you do. Don't worry about running a specific distance or feel pressure to enter a race. Feel good about whatever you are able to do, and make a commitment to continue.

Create a habit. The discipline to stick with a schedule and alter your activity habits is extremely important, but sometimes it takes a while to develop. It's natural to experience some difficulty during the first month or so, but then it becomes gradually easier. So give yourself some time and don't expect miracles overnight. Remember – you're seeking long-term results.

Find a friend. One of the key factors in maintaining any exercise program is having someone to exercise with. It can be your spouse, your child, a work acquaintance, or some random stranger you meet at a group run. Having an exercise partner makes you accountable, and helps pass the time during workouts. Best of all, before too long, that relative stranger may become a good friend.

Have fun! Running shouldn't be drudgery. Training time is playtime. Think of it as recess from your daily grind.

Dr. George Sheehan was a modern-day running philosopher who once wrote, "Heed the inner calling to your own play … you can reawaken the passion, relive the dream, and recapture your youth." We couldn't agree with him more; running makes us feel like kids on a playground, every single day.

So … NOW do you think you can start running?

Dr. Sheehan also wrote, "My fitness program was a campaign, a revolution, a conversion. I was determined to find myself. In the process, I found my body and the soul that went with it." We want our readers to have similar conversions, and find themselves the exact same way.

Go Team!

GO TEAM! If you make a habit of running or watching marathons, you'll hear spectators and runners yelling this cheer loudly and consistently from start to finish.

The cheers are meant as encouragement for the countless runners in purple Team in Training (TNT) singlets – but their larger meaning is so much more.

Team in Training is the world's largest endurance sports coaching program, which provides training for individuals to participate in half or full marathons, triathlons, cycling events, adventure races, or cross-country skiing events. They cater primarily to beginner athletes who would never imagine completing one of these tasks alone.

But the races are not the main emphasis. They are tools that allow thousands of people each year to raise money for the Leukemia and Lymphoma Society.

Their distinctive purple shirts started appearing at marathons in 1988. Since then about 300,000 people have trained with TNT and raised almost 700 million dollars for research towards a cure for leukemia, lymphoma, Hodgkin's disease, and myeloma, as well as improving the quality of life of patients and their families.

TNT runners receive personalized fitness training, workouts, and clinics by certified coaches for a period of four or five months, a supportive group of teammates to train with, and lodging and airfare to the event of their choice. Many previous TNT runners stay involved with the group as mentors and captains.

There are more than 60 accredited events in the United States and overseas. The typical amount required for fund raising is in the $2,500 to $4,000 range, depending on how exotic the event location is. Participants receive a fundraising website and prepared material to help as well.

On race day, they get the purple shirt and all of those encouraging yells.

TNT participants come from various backgrounds. Most are trying their first-ever athletic event. About 75% are women. The average age is 37. About 25% are TNT alumni doing another event. An impressive 99% of those who make it to the starting line of their event are able to finish the race.

Although the emphasis is fundraising, the coaches emphasize fitness and fun and healthy lifestyle changes. There are clinics on nutrition, injury prevention, race strategy, and running form. Each person meets an "honored teammate," who is a local cancer survivor whose own courage provides inspiration and motivation.

TNT's popularity continues to grow. In large cities like San Francisco, Los Angeles, or New York, you might see hundreds of team participants running together on Saturday mornings in preparation for their next event. In smaller towns you have to look a bit harder, but there are usually groups of at least five or six locals who run together.

Topher Mueller, team captain and mentor for the Monterey Peninsula region, says the key is the group encouragement and support. He notes that people join for many reasons. Most are from families that have been touched by leukemia or lymphoma. Many run to honor a friend or relative. Some are just seeking a healthier lifestyle and want to start a fitness program with the support of a group environment which also happens to have a charity component.

TNT is a win-win situation for everyone involved. Novice runners become involved in running, cycling, or triathlon while raising funds to fight devastating diseases. Races appreciate having large groups of dedicated, enthusiastic participants at their events. And millions of people who battle these serious diseases benefit from the research and treatment breakthroughs this fundraising supports.

Our hope for those runners is that when they complete their big event, they don't consider it the final finish line. Marathons or triathlons shouldn't just be something to check off of life's "to do" list, and TNT provides a fantastic opportunity to develop a running or fitness program to be maintained for life. We wish their participants continued success in all of their future athletic and charitable endeavors.

And GO TEAM!!!

Take 5 to Run

Over the years we have written numerous columns lamenting the obesity problem that plagues America. Unfortunately, the last 30 years of public service announcements, nutritional education, and instruction on physical activity has done little to curb the epidemic, as both children and adults are still getting fatter.

This time we're taking a different approach: it's a call to action, and we're encouraging all of our running friends to get involved. It's time to stop talking about the issue, and start DOING something about it.

If you're like us, you know how great running makes you feel, both physically and mentally. You know how beneficial it is for your cardiovascular health and emotional wellbeing. You also know how rewarding it feels to share these experiences with others.

So here's what we want you to do: participate in an effort called Take 5 to Run. It's not really an official program; in fact, we just made it up. But the premise is quite simple, and has the potential to be highly effective.

Look at the numbers. There are currently 30 million adults who claim they run at least a few times a month. 10 million of them run "regularly" and entered organized races last year. These are the people whom we're asking to Take 5 to Run.

Over the course of one year, invite 5 of your non-running friends for a run. Encourage them to get started, help them to select shoes or other gear if needed, and take them on an easy jog. Help them through the initial uncertainty, and celebrate every accomplishment on their way to starting a running program.

Later, ask them to pay it forward; once they are established runners, recommend that they take another 5 people out for a run. And so on and so on. Do the math: if 10 million runners recruit 50 million non-runners, and that group grows to 250 million in a couple of years … before you know it we have a nation of runners and the obesity trend is reversed.

Obviously, we aren't naive enough to think that everyone will successfully convert 5 others, but we optimistically believe that many of you are capable of drawing new runners in. As long as the numbers trend in the right direction, we'll still end the epidemic. So how do you instruct someone to start? Remember the name of the game.

Take 5 to Run is a phrase that can also be used as a blueprint to get friends or kids started. The first run or walk should only be 5 minutes. Aim for a habit of 5 minutes per day, 5 days a week. Tell 5 people about it, for moral support and to hold yourself accountable. Select one day to increase your distance by 5 more minutes, and then another day, and then another and another as you continue to improve.

We'd also love to see the running industry step up and help people Take 5 to Run. Shoe companies or specialty running stores could give discounts to those who say they are buying their first pair of shoes and mention Take 5 to Run. Races should give discounts to those who are entering their first race after they've Taken 5 to Run. Get some national running organizations on board, and who knows where this might end up.

But for the time being, it can all begin with you. Take the pledge, and Take 5 to Run.

Long May You Run

If you learn only one thing from reading our columns on a regular basis, we hope it is this: running and physical activity will enrich your life in numerous ways, at any age.

We frequently talk about the rewards of getting youngsters involved in running. The current generation of children is a generation in crisis, because of childhood obesity and many other health risks.

I (Mike) have attended many national seminars on childhood obesity, and they often use the same opening quote: "This generation of children will be the first generation in history to live shorter lives than their parents." Any parent or grandparent can attest that this is certainly a frightening prospect.

But it doesn't have to be this way. As an optimistic elder member of the baby boomer generation I want to consider the opposite scenario.

What if, instead of watching our descendents live shorter life spans, we swing the pendulum all the way to the other extreme? Let's make the next generation the first one to measure life spans in centuries rather than years. It's a possibility that's not that far-fetched.

Scientific advances and future breakthroughs in medical research have the potential to optimize disease prevention and medical treatment, increasing the longevity of humans many decades longer than we currently imagine. The future could be one crazy place – just consider the following example.

Look in the crystal ball to the year 2106. It's the 121st annual Big Sur Marathon. The race entry fee has become enormous; somewhat because of inflation, but mostly because of an increased budget due to all the age group awards. There are 50,000 people running in several waves because virtually everyone in 2106 is a runner. It's one of the reasons for increased longevity.

There is fierce competition in the 140 to 144-year-old category for the 5 age group awards provided. I hear one competitor saying, "It seems like the same guys that beat me when I was only 102 are still beating me! I can hardly wait to turn 145 so I'll be in a new age category."

Another 173-year-old competitor comments, "I hate it that my times are so much slower than when I was in my 160's. What I'd give to be that young again."

Fantastical and absurd? I don't think so.

Back to the present day. For many years, I've taught training clinics to help new runners prepare for the Big Sur Marathon. During the first session, I always trot in runners from the previous year who have successfully trained and completed their first marathon. They describe to the wary participants how running Big Sur was one of the greatest experiences of their lives. They admit their own initial fears and explained how they overcame them to train properly and finish the race.

I always try to showcase a wide variety of runners in order to instill confidence in the newbies. A few years back I invited a 74-year-old man who didn't start running until he was 72 and completed his first Big Sur Marathon the following year.

He was very pleased to come and talk to the group. He spoke eloquently about his experience and answered every question from the rapt audience.

But after the session he came up to me and said, "You invited me because I am a freak."

Although I didn't want to, I had to confess that he was basically right. That is *exactly* why I invited him. If younger runners see someone much older finishing the marathon it immediately makes them think they can also do it.

I also told him that to non-runners, anyone who runs is a freak – and anyone who runs a marathon is certifiable. To most runners however, it is a pretty common sight to see 60-, 70-, or occasionally even 80-year-olds at the start of a marathon. This year's Big Sur Marathon had 14 finishers who were 70 years or older. Another 97 runners were between 60 and 69.

I definitely considered my guest speaker an ATHLETE and not a freak.

Don't just wait for future medical breakthroughs. You can take charge of your own health right now. You too can become an athlete. Just get out there and run, or do something else that makes you physically active.

How would you like people to describe you as you grow older - as a couch potato or an athlete? Do you want to be a role model to those who follow you, or an example of behaviors to avoid? Those types of decisions should be easy ones, no matter what age you are, or how many more years you have remaining.

Go ahead and get started. You'll find lots of help along the way.

ROAD-TESTED ADVICE

"Most runners become amazingly adept at recognizing their friends from a long distance away by their unique running styles. Even in the dark, a distinctive bounce or arm swing or posture or tilt of the head gives everyone away. Running styles become your own personal signature, almost like a fingerprint."

"In order to run faster, you have to train faster (well, duh). The tricky part is learning how to do this without getting hurt. Here, then, are our Top Gun Rules of Engagement for transforming your 747 body into an F-16."

Snot Rocket Science

(Warning: the following column contains graphic descriptions of an unflattering body function. Make sure you've finished breakfast before reading.)

During the winter months, there's an easy way to spot the novices in a crowd of runners: they're the ones carrying Kleenex.

The rest of us, after enough training miles, eventually become skilled in the delicate practice of clearing our nasal passages using nothing more than one finger and a well-timed blast of air. Today, we're going to explain how it's done.

That's right ... we're talking about snot rockets.

Runners certainly didn't invent the process of ejecting snot directly onto the ground, but – like everything else we do – we've trained ourselves to do it very efficiently. In the wintertime, the combination of cold temperatures and lingering congestion force many runners to become experts in the technique.

The act is also known as "farmer blowing," but this moniker doesn't accurately reflect the amount of skill and risk that are involved in the procedure. It's not exactly rocket science, but it's fairly complicated nevertheless ... so let's just call it snot rocket science.

Yes, there is risk involved, and several factors to consider in order to launch these projectiles safely. So follow this advice, and no one gets hurt.

The first lesson in snot rocketry is timing. You can't just run out the front door and start blasting. The human nostril is a complex mechanism, with narrow parameters of operational efficiency. The machinery needs proper lubrication to perform effectively, a process that can take several minutes after the start of your run. If you try to launch from a dry chamber, you're bound to just push the payload down onto your cheek.

You also have to wait until your snot reaches the proper critical mass for expulsion. The test is to exhale gently through your nose, and if you feel substantive thickness and pressure on the rim of your nostril, you know that all systems are go.

However, before launching, you need to carefully check your surroundings. A typical rocket travels downward with a posterior and lateral trajectory – think of a cone-shaped distribution range – so you shouldn't be alongside or in front of other runners when you let fly. Proper etiquette dictates that a runner moves well off to the side of a group, to ensure that his/her fellow runners remain out of the blast line. Be sure to check your blind spot over your shoulder as well to avoid any friendly fire incidents.

Another consideration if you're running in a public place is to check that there aren't any impressionable children – or anyone else who might be offended – around when you blow. Rocket launching is similar to swearing: generally OK for grown-ups to do under certain circumstances, but not something you want kids to go around mimicking without understanding the ramifications.

Once you've determined the proper launch time and assured your positioning, it's time to pay attention to technique. There's nothing more embarrassing than coming home with a giant booger on your shoulder or thigh because of a sloppy misfire.

(Before we proceed further, here's one final disclaimer: Please note that the following instructions pertain to unilateral [one-sided] launching. The method of discharging both nostrils simultaneously – sometimes referred to as a Double Texan – is a highly risky maneuver to be attempted only by experienced practitioners.)

It isn't as simple as turning your head and blowing. The recommended technique for single-nostril blasting is to rotate your shoulders and hips slightly to the "involved" side, leaning partially forward from the waist. Inhale slowly while placing the pad of your index or middle finger beside the opposite (non-rocket) nostril. Gently press the nostril shut while you forcefully exhale, expulsing the contents of the full nostril onto the ground.

Some runners prefer the European variation of hand positioning, where the pad of the thumb is placed upon the opposite nostril, with the remaining fingers extended above the blast line. While this is an acceptable alternative, the gesture is sometimes viewed as more offensive in nature, and the finger-on-nose technique is generally recognized as the gold standard.

Once the projectile has launched, there's probably some cleanup work to be done. Even if you have a clean shoot, most rockets will leave some splatter residue when they exit the blast chamber. After a successful launch, check to see if you need to wipe any such debris from the base of your nose or the margins of your upper lip.

Pay attention when wiping, however, and be certain to maintain adequate separation of wiping surfaces. Many runners use the tips of their gloves or the sleeve of their shirt to wipe sweat off their foreheads while running. When clearing away rocket residue, use a different section of your garments, and then – this is the important part – remember which parts of your clothing you're using to wipe sweat, and which you're using to wipe snot. You'll feel like an idiot – not to mention look pretty gross – if you remove the stuff from your nose only to smear it around on your forehead a few minutes later.

Who knew there was so much to learn about blowing your nose? We don't call it snot rocket science for nothing. The good news is that most runners become proficient in the technique after a handful of practice sessions.

And once they do, they don't have to worry about bringing Kleenex on their training runs ever again.

The Circle Back

Here's a common problem many runners encounter: if two people want to run together, but their speed is significantly different, is there any way for them to be compatible?

The short answer is, yes – if it's done properly. But there are some guidelines that must be adhered to. Believe it or not, this topic has been thoroughly examined among our running group, and adherence to the guidelines has possibly saved some marriages and preserved friendships between runners of different speeds. (Honestly - we're not exaggerating as much as you think.)

So what's the magic solution? Our answer to the problem of pace incompatibility is known as the "circle back," where the faster runner will run ahead for a period of time, then retrace his or her steps to rejoin the other person a short while later.

It's a simple premise - but unfortunately, it's fraught with psychological landmines as one or both people may get their feelings hurt, or feel that the shared workout wasn't worthwhile. That's where the ground rules come in; follow these tips, and no one gets offended:

1. The faster runner always gives advance notice. "Stay comfortable, I'll circle back" is a good phrase to use before surging ahead. Sometimes, the circleback location can be agreed upon, but this is not an imperative.
2. The faster person breaks clean and runs ahead – typically to the top of a climb, a fork in the trail, or simply until feeling "worked out" - then doubles back toward the slower person, or runs out and back on a side trail or road until meeting up with the slower person again.
3. The faster runner returns to the main trail <u>behind</u> the slower runner and gradually matches the pace to allow resumption of conversation.

4. When rejoining the slower person, the faster runner should never, EVER make witty comments about the slower runner's pace. Trust us – your best-intentioned remark is sure to be interpreted as a put-down. Don't even make eye contact with the slower person, which may be interpreted as demeaning.
5. Don't give the slower person advice. Don't give him a phony complement. This is the most delicate part of the entire process, so be very cautious. If in doubt, just shut up and keep running. The slower person will talk when he's ready. (As an added caution, the aforementioned rule is twice as important if your slower running partner happens to be your spouse. Take our word for it.)

The circle back process can be repeated as many times as desired during the course of a run. But as a general rule, the fewer times it happens, the lower the risk of interpersonal tension.

There's another variation to this theory, which is kind of an inverse circle back. Occasionally, a faster runner will allow the slower runner to run ahead, while they hang back for some equipment adjustment (such as tying shoelaces or taking off a jacket), or "biological adjustment" (a bathroom break). Sometimes the stop is legitimate, other times not. If you're the slower runner, don't question it – just keep running, and be thankful for the company when the faster runner returns.

The circle back theory is versatile enough to be proper etiquette for larger groups of runners as well. The main idea is that with a little flexibility, everyone can enjoy each other's company, and each runner can still have a satisfying workout.

If it helps you maintain a friendship or avoid an argument with your spouse, so much the better. The next time you're with a group of runners, feel free to employ the circle back!

Lessons from the Sunday Weigh-In

There are no secrets at the Sunday Weigh-In.

In April of 1990, one of our running partners surprised everyone by pulling a scale out of his car after our regular Sunday morning run. About a dozen of us weighed in, and the numbers were recorded.

The weigh-in has continued nearly every week since then. We now have 15 years of recorded weights from over 100 runners, which also provide some insight about the runner's approach to weight management.

With overwhelming consistency, we have seen that each member of our group has about a 10-pound weight fluctuation throughout the year. Each of them are typically fastidious, well aware of their weight on any given day, and whether they are heavier or lighter than usual.

What separates runners from "cosmetic" dieters is that we tend to have better volitional control over our weight, and can change it in a relatively short period of time. In the weeks leading up to a marathon, almost everybody in the group trends downward toward the bottom of their weight range. Our weekly weigh-in data has taught us that we've all run our fastest marathons when running at our lowest weights.

So how do runners lose an extra 10 pounds when they need to? We don't spend money on self-help weight loss books. We don't depend on trendy diets (and we're all rejoicing the long-overdue death of the Atkins fad). We don't restrict ourselves to single food groups or eliminate pleasure foods.

The secret of our group is rather simple: when we need to lose weight, we just eat less and run more.

That's it. That's all there is. We couldn't write a book and make money on this premise because the explanation is way too short. The plain truth is that your weight is primarily determined by the ratio of calories in to calories out. It really isn't any more complicated than that.

On the "calories out" side, a conventional rule is that you burn about 100 calories per mile, regardless of speed. Therefore, running 8 miles will burn approximately 800 total calories.

Research indicates that a speed of 5 miles per hour is necessary for this guideline to be applicable, which equates to a 12-minute mile; it's a very brisk walking speed, but a somewhat leisurely jogging pace.

Your body also burns a certain amount of calories per day just to function normally – for most people, about 2,000 calories, give or take a couple hundred. Regular exercise increases the caloric expenditure above that baseline level. While it is theoretically possible to lose weight without exercising, your practical chance of success is virtually nonexistent.

Now look at some examples of "calories in." A Starbucks grande caffe mocha without whipped cream contains about 300 calories. With non-fat milk it's down to 220, which requires about 2 miles of running to burn off. Include a blueberry scone with its 460 calories, and you've added nearly 5 miles of running to balance the ratio.

Stop for a McDonald's quarter pounder with cheese (510 calories) or a Taco Bell bean burrito (370 calories) on your lunch break, and soon you'll need to run all day long just to break even.

Alcoholic beverages are notoriously loaded with calories, as a 4-ounce glass of wine has about 100 calories and a 12-ounce beer has 150 calories. Desserts are obviously dangerous, too – a single scoop of ice cream will cost you about three miles of running. That doesn't mean you can't have these treats, but you'll have to cut back on something else that day.

Obviously some foods have better health benefits than others, but at the end of the day, weight loss basically hinges on burning more calories than you take in. Following this concept while enjoying everything in moderation makes weight management remarkably simple.

Our group of runners aren't calorie-counters, but we're all aware of these guidelines. When we want to lose weight, we either ramp up our mileage (and calories burned) or decrease our food consumption. We know there are times to "heat up the furnace" and increase the burn when preparing for a race, and other times when we can ease off a bit. We don't worry about small fluctuations in our weight because we know we can get it under control when necessary.

Even if you're not an endurance athlete, adopting the runner's approach to nutrition is an easy way to manage your weight. And if you ever run with us on a Sunday morning, don't be surprised to see the scale waiting for you when you're finished.

The Barefoot Renaissance

"The human foot is a masterpiece of engineering and a work of art."

- Leonardo da Vinci

We're on record several times claiming that running is the simplest sport in the world, because all you need is a pair of shoes.

However, a steadily growing contingent of runners is determined to prove that notion incorrect. Not the part about the simplicity – the part about needing shoes.

Barefoot running is nothing new, of course – it dates back many millennia before the waffle sole launched Nike into the stratosphere. Some anthropologists believe our prehistoric ancestors were tremendous runners, hunting animals by chasing them to the point of exhaustion. It makes sense if you do the math: hominids were on Earth 6 million years ago, but mankind's first known weapons are only about 500,000 years old. So unless all those cavemen were vegetarians, they must have had some means of catching and killing prey.

Even in the modern era, barefoot runners have competed at world-class levels. Abebe Bikila won a gold medal and set a world record in the 1960 Olympic marathon. Zola Budd is notorious (to American fans, at least) for her collision with Mary Decker at the 1984 Los Angeles Olympics, but she also won back to back world cross-country championships in the

1980s. A handful of ultrarunners often run barefoot on mountain trails to complement their high mileage training routines.

You may think that this is terrible for your feet – but the truth might be exactly the opposite. There's currently a philosophical war raging among shoe manufacturers: on one side are the folks who think that foot asymmetries and irregularities should be corrected by various means of support and motion control. The other side believes that less is more; if you allow the foot to work naturally, the irregularities don't matter. Not only that, but overcorrecting the foot's natural motion actually leads to higher injury rates.

Think of it this way: if you were engineering the perfect weight bearing structure, you'd create an arch. For optimal shock absorption, you'd allow that arch to flex slightly upon impact. For dynamic energy transfer, you'd surround it with several interlocking components that move in multiple directions. For durability, you'd make the building blocks out of the hardest material you can create.

Well, guess what you've just designed? The human foot! 26 bones and 33 joints crafted together to form an anatomical arch, held together by more than 100 muscles, tendons, and ligaments all working in harmony. And yet, for the better part of 40 years, the prevailing philosophy within the running shoe industry was that this particular part of the human body was somehow created imperfectly, so they turned to technology to fix it.

Consequently, shoe companies' mission over the past few decades was to augment the apparent shortcomings of natural biomechanics. They cushioned our heelstrike with air pillows or gel chambers or elastic grids. They prevented our pronation with rollbars and medial posts. They limited our ankle motion with stability devices or rigid platforms. And since modern runners are constantly told that they need specialized shoes to prevent injury, they've come to rely on these devices to keep them running comfortably from one year to the next.

Barefoot runners believe that from a biomechanical standpoint, there's really no reason you need to wear shoes, and that the shoe industry is trying to fix something – the structure and function of the human foot – that wasn't broken to begin with. With increasing numbers, traditional runners are starting to listen, but they often find that barefoot running is more challenging than they bargained for.

The primary drawbacks are comfort and speed. Running barefoot is certainly uncomfortable right off the bat; our feet aren't used to the lack of artificial cushioning, and our skin needs time to build resiliency to irritants like gravel, sticks, and pointy rocks. In order to accommodate these, the runner is forced to slow down much more than he's normally accustomed to.

Most of us aren't patient enough to put up with it – but the drumbeat of barefoot runners is growing ever louder; so much, in fact, that the entire shoe industry has taken notice.

The Vibram company, better known for supplying outsoles to traditional shoe manufacturers, makes a brilliant product called Five Fingers, which is basically a glove for your foot with a thin rubber coating underneath. The added protection effectively allows you to run barefoot without worrying about injuring yourself on broken glass or rusty nails. Several small companies are moving into the "minimalist" category, with models that are little more than a foot covering and an outsole. More tellingly, many heavyweights such as Nike, New Balance, ECCO, and Terra Plana now have models that promote the natural biomechanics of running with naked feet. It appears that the barefoot revolution has successfully carved out an entirely new (and growing) niche in the footwear industry.

However, there's one important caveat to all this: whether you're running barefoot or in minimalist shoes, you have to progress extremely slowly. Your normal form and body mechanics will be significantly altered, and your lower leg muscles need a very long time to adapt to all the changes. If you impatiently try to do too much mileage too soon, you'll end up extremely sore and at even greater risk of injury than when you started.

When it comes to what kind of shoes – if any – to put on your feet, there really isn't any 100% correct answer. Some runners thrive on going shoeless, while others will run for decades in traditional footwear without any problems at all. From our standpoint, as long as everybody is running, there's really no need to worry about which side is right.

Donald Buraglio and Michael Dove

Let's Talk About Sex

"Let's talk about sex, baby –

Let's talk about you and me –

Let's talk about all the good things and the bad things that may be."

– Salt 'n' Pepa, "Let's Talk about Sex"

It's perhaps one of the most contentious questions ever asked: does sex affect your athletic performance? For as long as people have played games, there has been disagreement as to whether those other kinds of "games" are a help or a hindrance.

During the 4th century BC, Plato described the training regimen of Ikkos of Tarentum leading up to the ancient Olympic Games. According to Jane Spencer of the *Wall Street Journal*, Ikkos was a legendary athlete who was known to consume large quantities of cheese and goat meat, and often rubbed his skin with olive oil to make his muscles gleam. He also gave up sex during his peak training buildup (not too surprising, really, considering that olive oil thing), and went on to win the Olympic Pentathlon. Plato's account is considered the first documented endorsement of abstinence before competition.

However, famed historian Pliny the Elder turned the argument on its head in his best-selling (or whatever they called something that was popular back then) treatise *Natural History*, released in AD 77. Pliny's statement that "Athletes when sluggish are revitalized by love-making" was like an Emancipation Proclamation for horny athletes everywhere.

The battle has raged ever since. While most studies show that getting busy causes no tangible difference in athletic performance, athletes in all sports have weighed in on both sides. When it comes to shagging, it seems that everyone has something to say.

American track star Marty Liquori was one of the first runners to promote abstinence before races, saying that he liked to be "angry and aggressive" to race a fast mile. He explained that, "If you've had sex the night before, you'll be in a satisfied state and feel like smoking a cigarette." Victor Plata, a member of the U.S. Olympic triathlon team, took the angry and aggressive approach to the extreme; Plata says he went 233 days without tapping, becoming "completely monastic" before the 2004 Athens Olympics.

However, in Olympic competition, it's very likely that both Liquori and Plata were defeated by competitors who got their freak on just before the event. Among athletes, the Olympic Village is one of the most sexually vigorous gatherings imaginable. Whenever thousands of hardbodies with boundless energy and excess time on their hands gather together, the results are highly predictable.

At the Albertville Winter Games, condom machines in the athletes' village reportedly had to be refilled every two hours. In Sydney, the organizers' original order of 70,000 condoms was drained so quickly that they had to order 20,000 more - and the supply was still exhausted three days before the end of competition.

Breaux Greer, an American javelin thrower at the Sydney Games, reported that "There's a LOT of sex going on. You get people who are in shape, and testosterone's up, and everybody's attracted to everybody." Such thoughts give new meaning to the concept of international diplomacy.

And yet, athletes continue to have differences of opinion on the effects of bedroom tapering. British sprinter Linford Christie habitually refrained, saying that a romp the night before a race made his legs feel like lead. On the other hand, the great Bob Beamon once reported that he got some action on the eve of his record-shattering long jump at the 1968 Mexico City Olympics. Christie won one Olympic gold medal in the 100 meters, but Beamon set a world record that stood for 23 years. Draw your own conclusions.

Noted baseball sage Casey Stengel had an interesting take on the matter. Stengel liked to say that being with a woman never hurt a baseball player – it was the staying up all night to look for a woman that did him in. So presumably, if a willing partner just happened to be lying in the same bed, Stengel would give his players the green light.

Finally, Brazilian soccer star Ronaldo claimed that the key to his success in winning the 2002 World Cup was getting his groove on just before each match. He also says that to save his strength, he let his wife do most of the work. The lesson here is … actually, we're not really sure there is a lesson here – we just thought it was a great story.

So the professionals are clearly undecided. But what about recreational athletes? Does boinking more frequently make us better competitors? Or conversely, does being a runner help you have a great sex life? None of us is trying to set any world records, but if a little extra bumping and grinding would help our race results, that would be good news indeed.

First - to set the record straight - we make no claim to be authorities in this field. Although we know a lot about training, we don't pretend to have any expertise in knocking boots. We can, however, give you some opinions and anecdotes from local runners, and allow you to make your own decisions.

For instance, one of our running partners is a respected physician who says he always thinks about sex while running, and likewise thinks about running whenever he's exercising horizontally. He insists that it makes both his running and his sex life better. However, we're keeping his identity anonymous so that he remains respected.

Another of our local marathon runners also happens to be an instructor of human sexuality at CSU –Monterey Bay. She says the safest and most effective method for increasing your sex drive is proper diet and exercise. Running develops an enhanced cardiovascular system, with increased blood flow to ALL parts of the body. Therefore, running may affect your sex drive as much as boffing affects your running performance.

Additionally, consider a series of recent studies – some funded by Pfizer Inc., makers of Viagra - which indicate that regular sexual activity boosts levels of testosterone, one of the prime hormonal agents responsible for athletic performance in both men and women. Researchers found that sustained testosterone levels rose markedly when participants of either gender began having sex regularly.

(2008 addendum: now that we think of it ... maybe Floyd Landis didn't cheat in the Tour de France after all - maybe he just got a TON of French hospitality the night before that crucial mountain stage. How come no one else thought of this defense?)

Sex and running ... running and sex. No matter what your personal preferences for pre-race competition may be, these topics will inevitably continue to be joined at the hip (so to speak) for countless years to come.

So what about our own personal experience? Are you wondering how often we get sprung, and what it does for our running? Honestly, we'd love to tell you. We're always willing to share our knowledge, and we've said many times that there are no secrets in running.

Unfortunately, our wives DO keep some secrets. And on this particular subject, that's all we're allowed to say.

Look Down

"Look up. Look down. Look at my thumb..."

Remember the end of this joke from when you were a kid? That's what we're talking about this week – except we're leaving out the part about you being dumb. For now, think of it as a mantra to remember good running form, and to have fun or learn something while doing it.

Conventional wisdom says you should keep your eyes straight ahead while running. However, the two of us are anything but conventional – so here is our own advice, based on the aforementioned joke.

First, for proper form, try to **look at your thumbs** while you run.

Keep your hands loosely closed with thumbs pointing up at about a 45 degree angle toward the midline of your body. Pretend you are holding an egg in your hands to avoid clenching. This relaxed position will translate to your forearms, shoulders, and neck, which will help your body run more efficiently.

Now for the fun parts – that's where **looking up** and **looking down** come in handy. Some of our most memorable running experiences have come when we let our eyes wander above and below, as the following examples show.

Look down: to find money! Areas like subdivisions or commercial districts often have all sorts of spare change lying in the roads or sidewalks. Shopping mall parking lots are great for finding coins – just be sure to look up every now and then to avoid cars.

Sure, it's not exactly a gold mine out there – what you find is usually just a dime or a few pennies – but over the course of 20 years or so, you might save enough to buy a can of soda someday. Either that, or just do what we do: put the change in our kids' and grandkids' piggy banks.

Look up: and gaze upon the heavens at night. See the stars and planets, and look for space shuttles, satellites, space stations, meteor showers, and other celestial objects. If you have a friend who's an astronomer, take him running with you one night; trust us, you'll learn more than you ever imagined.

Look down: for sporting goods – especially around local country clubs. If you ever need used tennis balls for playing fetch with your dog, just run around the perimeter of a tennis club sometime. We've found dozens of balls over the years while running around the courts, and usually thrown them back over the fence. We just hope the golfers there have better aim than the tennis players.

Look up: for birds of prey. As the dawn breaks on local trails, we frequently see owls, hawks, and vultures. Seeing vultures when you are tired and thirsty and a long way from home is somewhat disconcerting – but it's an impressive sight nevertheless.

Look down: for mile markers. Many commonly used roads have cryptic markings in chalk or spray paint, sometimes with strange initials near them. Some of these are from local races, or from neighborhood runners marking their regular courses. These are helpful to judge your pace during routine workouts.

We have both run in the Las Vegas desert west of the Strip, following the old LVM (Las Vegas Marathon) mile markers, which made for a nice occasional distraction from the dust and the tumbleweeds.

Look up: for architecture. Running in an urban downtown area is a great way to take in the design and decorative features of historic buildings. You'd be surprised at how many gargoyles there are, in places you wouldn't expect.

Look down: for history. Historical markers are abundant on city streets. Mike often runs in San Francisco near AT&T Park, and one day noticed a large bronze plaque marked *Rammaytush*. Initially, he had no idea what it could possibly mean – until he gave himself a history lesson.

It turns out that Rammaytush is the name of an indigenous people native to the Mission district of San Francisco. The word is from a combined dialect of the Mitsun people and the Awaswas. Their language consisted of only 173 words, and each one is embedded in a sidewalk in the city, along with its English translation.

Perhaps the strangest and most famous street markings are the "smoots" on the Harvard Bridge over the Charles River between Boston and Cambridge. The smoot is a distance measure named after Oliver Smoot of the MIT class of 1962. Smoot was a fraternity pledge who was used by his brothers to measure the bridge. One smoot is equal to Oliver's height (five feet seven inches), and he repeatedly lay down on the bridge so his classmates could mark each unit in paint.

The bridge's official length was determined to be "364.4 smoots plus one ear." Today, anyone running across the bridge can still see the painted smoot markings, thanks to the incoming fraternity pledges who repaint them each year.

It's also interesting to footnote that Oliver Smoot later became the President of the International Organization for Standardization and recently retired as chairman of the American National Standards Institute. Today's Google calculator even uses smoots as an optional unit of measure.

And you might not have known that if you weren't reading this column about running. There's a whole world of fascinating things you can learn as a runner, even more if you remember to look up and down.

Introduction to Trail Running

Trail running is one of the great pleasures in our sport. There is absolutely no feeling that compares to cruising through a dense oak forest, alongside a rippling stream, or high atop a mountain ridge. Experienced runners appreciate the many benefits of trail running, and incorporate it into their year-round training. When summer approaches, the number of people on the trails increases, as long daylight hours allows early morning or evening users to join the fun.

For the novice trail runner, we are discussing proper preparation for heading off the beaten path. For experienced users, we are reviewing basic trail etiquette so that everyone can enjoy the trails responsibly.

Preparation for trail running

Weather: Temperatures on the trail can run to extremes: dangerously warm in the summer, and extremely cold in the winter. Your preparations need to be more extensive as well; bring extra fluids in warm weather, and wear extra clothes for the cold. If the weather is unpredictable, dress in layers so you're ready for anything.

Use a map: There are no street signs in the parks, and not every footpath is identified, so it's easy to get disoriented and take off in the wrong direction. And unlike city streets, it's not easy to correct a mistake. Taking a wrong turn on a trail could easily turn a 45-minute jog into a 2-hour ordeal.

Most parks have maps available at the main entrances, so you can grab one to carry with you on your way in. If you don't know the area (or if you can't read a map), run with a buddy who knows the trails well.

Know the trails: You not only need to know where the trails go, but what the terrain is like. The shortest line on your map isn't always the fastest route. A narrow, rugged footpath can take considerably longer to traverse than a groomed fire road. Again, the buddy system is the best way to get acquainted with the terrain.

Hydrate: The increased heat and potential for long detours make it important to have water at your disposal. Most trail runners carry a small waist pack that holds a water bottle, keys, or even a small cell phone. Basic packs are available for $25-30, and are well worth the investment. For longer outings, consider a backpack-style hydration pack.

Watch for critters: In our years of trail running we have seen numerous coyotes, bobcats, wild turkeys, sheep, deer, raccoons, skunks and snakes. On rare occasions the more ominous mountain lion or wild boar may cross your path. Treat all of these creatures with respect – after all, you are intruding in their home. Encounters with critters are normally pleasant, but you should be aware of what to do in a threatening situation.

Shoes: Most shoe companies make specialized trail running shoes with such features as knobby tread, water-resistant uppers, and lower heel angles (to improve the base of support). However, these are largely unnecessary unless you are logging high mileage on challenging trails. Your regular pair of running shoes should suffice, but our advice is to dedicate one pair of shoes to off-road use, and use another pair for the roads.

Trail etiquette

Right of way: Trails are shared by runners, hikers, mountain bikers, and equestrians. Many parks have signs indicating right of way for each, often depicted in a triangle graphic. Horses have the right of way at all times. Cyclists are supposed to yield to everybody, even dismounting if necessary. Runners have the right of way over bikes, but should yield to horses.

Approaching bikes: Although runners have right of way over bikers, usually the easiest solution on a narrow trail is for the runner to step off the trail and allow the bikes to pass. On a fire road, if approaching from opposite directions, the biker and runner should each move to the right.

If the biker comes up behind the runner, he should yell out a warning, then pass on the left while the runner moves right. (To clarify a point: if somebody shouts "On your left!" it means they are passing on your left side. The proper response for you is to move to the right. This seems obvious but often gets screwed up in practice.)

Approaching horses: Despite their large size, horses are actually prey animals whose instinct is to run when encountering unknown or frightening objects. Runners and bikers approaching horses from the front should stop and make sure the horse sees them, then proceed slowly to pass.

When approaching from the back, call out to the horse and rider to let them know you want to pass. Once you know the horse is aware of you and not startled, continue past them.

Usually the sound of a voice or the smell of a human is enough to reassure a horse that he's not in danger. Unfortunately, horses haven't quite evolved to the point of recognizing a screeching, fast moving, metallic-and-rubber-smelling mountain bike yet, so their first reaction is usually fear until the biker slows down and says something. Bikers, please use extra caution with the horses.

Leave it the way you found it: Imagine walking through a beautiful art exhibit, and seeing a pile of garbage in the middle of the hardwood floor. That's the same feeling trail runners get when coming across GU wrappers or discarded water bottles left by careless users.

Conscientious campers and hikers know to "pack out" whatever they bring into the wilderness, and the same rule applies to runners and bikers. Remember the old saying: take only pictures, leave only footprints!

The trails around your local area are fantastic resources for everyone to enjoy. With a little preparation and common courtesy, trail running will become a valuable addition to your overall training regimen. Once you get started on the trails, you may find it difficult to return to running on the roads.

A Runner's Letter to Santa

TO: Santa Claus

LOCATION: North Pole

Dear Santa,

How are you doing? I know you're awfully busy this week, but I'm hoping you will have an extra minute to read this letter.

My friend Mike and I write a newspaper column about running and we sometimes give advice to runners preparing for races. Since you have a big event coming up, I thought you might appreciate some tips we have passed along to runners that are applicable to you also.

Actually Santa, you have more in common with runners than you might first suspect. You're probably aware that there are some people called ultramarathoners who also travel through the whole night, often running up to 30 or 40 consecutive hours. Ultrarunners and regular marathoners know the value of having the right gear to make a long task easier.

There are some great products out there that could make your job a lot easier. For instance, many runners use small LED headlamps when running in the dark. If you bought a set of eight for your reindeer you could see a lot better, you wouldn't be so dependent on Rudolph, and the extra lights would just be mistaken for stars in the sky. You get LL Bean catalogs up there, right? I got my headlamp from them, but many stores carry them as well.

A company called Garmin makes GPS units that tell you what altitude you are flying at, how many miles you have flown, and can give you global reference points so that you don't get lost. They're also pretty cool because they can tell you precisely how fast you are traveling, since I don't know if your sleigh has a working speedometer.

Another great gadget is a heart rate monitor (HRM) for your reindeer. Anytime you have a long run or trip it is important to pace yourself and not start out too quickly. HRMs are the best way to ensure this. I thought maybe you know about HRMs already, since the biggest manufacturer is called Polar. Are they based up near where you live?

When I run a marathon I keep my heart rate below 70% of my maximum for the first half of the race. If you strapped a HRM on each reindeer you could make sure they stay below 70% of their maximum heart rate in the Northern Hemisphere. I'm not sure what 70% of a reindeer's max HR would be, but there's probably a veterinarian on your list somewhere who could give you a reference chart, right? Then you can be sure your reindeer won't bonk somewhere over Patagonia.

Since you will be visiting several different parts of the world, it's important to dress in layers. And Santa, wool outerwear went out of fashion many years ago. You'd be far better off wearing a moisture-wicking base layer, some sort of performance fleece above it, with a water- and wind-resistant shell or parka as your outer layer.

The Under Armour company makes compression garments that are great base layers for outdoor activity. You may have seen them before, as they are similar to what Mr. Incredible wears when he goes out. They come in multiple colors, so you can keep wearing those red, white and black colors that you like. The other benefit you get from compression garments is that they give you a slimmer appearance by compressing your belly a little bit. I'll bet Mrs. Claus would like that, too.

Speaking of your gut, you should really work on getting rid of it during the off-season next year. I'm concerned about your long-term viability, Santa, for your well-being and for mine. In addition to all of the healthy benefits of losing weight, there would be room for more toys in the sleigh if you didn't occupy the whole front seat with your backside.

Plus, you could work a lot faster. Runners' conventional wisdom says that for every pound you lose, you can run an average mile 2 seconds faster. Figuring that you travel about 25,000 miles to circumnavigate the Earth, if you lost just 5 pounds, your reindeer could save 250,000 seconds of travel time pulling you across the sky.

Even factoring in the time you stop at each house, you could save enough time to return home and get a couple hours of sleep before those little elves come waking you up at the crack of dawn to show you the things they found under the tree that you already knew were there.

Think of your long night working as an endurance event, Santa – and as any good ultrarunner will tell you, during any long event it's important to keep taking in calories. I'm not really worried about you, because you've got about 100 million rest stops with cookies waiting at each one; I'm thinking again of your reindeer. Please make sure they stay hydrated and have some food during the trip. At my house I'll leave some Gatorade and CLIF Bars for you to give them - but don't worry, I'll still have cookies for you. Do you like chocolate chip? Those are my favorite.

Finally, there's one other matter I'd like to mention. My 4-year-old daughter (who I'm sure is on your "good" list) was considerate enough to ask for "running shoes for Daddy" on that list she sent you. I just wanted to clarify that I need men's size 11 trail running shoes. You can deliver them to the same address as the bag with the American Girl doll, the Leap Pad letterboard, and the slot car racing set.

My friend Mike celebrates Chanukah and he sometimes runs low on candles at this time of year, so when you swing by his house maybe you could drop some off to him. Don't get there too late, though, because he's usually awake by 4AM before he goes out running.

Thanks a lot Santa. Hopefully you'll find some of this information helpful on your trip this week. Have a Merry Christmas!

Sincerely,

Donald Buraglio

Carmel Valley, CA

The Need for Speed

In one of the most famous movie lines of the 1980s, Tom Cruise, playing a hot-shot pilot in *Top Gun*, says, "I feel the need…the need for SPEED!" Many runners, once they've experienced the excitement of entering a race, start to feel the same way. Just like Goose and Maverick, everyone wants to be faster.

Unfortunately, the need for speed is often a detriment to novice runners. And neither of us believes that speed work is necessary to obtain the many benefits of our sport. In training, you receive almost all the same healthy benefits from running slow as you do from running fast. However, since many runners are inherently competitive people, it is only natural that they want to learn to run faster.

So, one question we commonly hear is…"How do I get faster?"

The answer is quite simple: In order to run faster, you have to train faster (well, duh). The tricky part is learning how to do this without getting hurt. Here, then, are our Top Gun Rules of Engagement for transforming your 747 body into an F-16. For the next 700 words, think of us as Flight Instructors Jester and Viper. These rules aren't classified, so we won't even have to kill you after we tell you. Our operations manual is divided into three sections below:

Add speed play to your regular runs

Many runners think that they will improve and get faster by simply doing their routine training runs over and over, going a little bit faster each time. When you are a novice runner this is definitely true, as improvements in conditioning and strength will make your body more efficient, and gradually increase your base cruising speed. Unfortunately, it is only a matter of months before these improvements start to plateau. To continue improving, you need to place new stresses on your body. Speed play does this.

Start with what we call "striders," which are the best way to begin teaching your body to run faster without incurring any increased chance of injury.

Insert them into one of your regular daily runs instead of just running at your usual pace. After you have warmed up for at least one mile, start a 30-second strider this way: gradually speed up for about 10 seconds, sustain 15 seconds at that faster pace, then gradually slow down for the last 5 seconds until you are back to your regular pace. Don't stop after the strider, but continue along at your baseline pace.

When you feel completely rested and your breathing is back to normal, then do another strider. Start out with 4 or 5, and add one each week until you are doing 10 during your normal run. The speed of each strider should be the same, so they should feel reasonably comfortable, and never at 100% speed. You can also gradually stretch the period of time of each strider to 45 or 60 seconds.

After a few months of build up, you'll be ready for advanced flight instruction: training at the track. Track workouts have a whole different workout than regular training runs, so if you're new to the game, find a captain or wingman to show you the ropes.

Add Strength and Core Exercises

As Jester told Maverick, don't let your ego write checks that your body can't cash. If you want to train like the best of the best, you have to keep your equipment in good working order. Strength training is a great cross-training activity for runners, and helps to prevent injury while building speed. If you run every other day, then do strength training on your non-running days. If you run nearly every day, strength training should be done on your easy running days, and preferably at a different time of day (ie, two separate workouts).

We recommend strengthening both the legs and midsection. If you don't belong to a gym, it's not a problem; neither of us does either. There are many types of exercises that can be done at home on the floor or with very simple equipment. However, if you have never done strength training, we would recommend a coach or trainer for some initial guidance on correct technique.

There are many simple workouts (like physioballs or basic crunches) that primarily focus on the abdomen, or more systemic workouts like yoga and Pilates that also incorporate flexibility and breathing. Likewise, leg strengthening can be done by classic weight machines, or by plyometric activities like bounding or lateral jumping. Whatever types of exercise you choose, start gradually and build up slowly.

Be Patient

Building speed depends on multiple biomechanical and physiological adaptations developed over a long period of time. Progressing too quickly is the primary cause of injury in runners. If you are building up for a race, speed training has to be done over several months. Most runners measure their rates of improvement in years, not weeks. Trust us, the changes will come if you keep at it long enough.

Don't try to do too much at once. Excess speed work is the runner's equivalent of flying into the danger zone. Speed work should only be one small component of your overall training plan. If the percentage of overall training miles spent in speed training is too high, even experienced runners will start to break down with injuries.

Proper speed work is very effective in slashing minutes off of your race times, but it isn't child's play, and shouldn't be undertaken foolishly. Remember, the Top Gun Rules of Engagement are written for your safety, and the safety of your training partners. So when you get the urge to turn and burn, just remember to follow the rules so that nobody gets hurt.

Taper Time

Tapering is a period of "active rest" when your body recovers from all those weeks of hard training. It's the delicate balance between running and resting that brings you to the starting line fresh and ready to go. Tapering is especially critical in the weeks leading up to running a marathon.

The process is tricky. If you run too much, you'll be overly tired on the starting line. If you rest too much, you won't feel sharp on race day, and may not run as effectively as possible.

In other words, there are lots of ways to screw things up. So we've compiled out best advice for tapering before your big event to maximize your chance of race day success.

No more long runs: Your final long run should be no less than 14 days before the marathon. If you've missed some of your scheduled long runs, it's too late to make up for it now. Anything above 15 miles will most likely hurt your performance on race day.

Cut back the mileage: Decrease your total weekly mileage by about 40% in the upcoming week. During race week, reduce your overall mileage by at least 60%. For example, a runner whose weekly training mileage peaked at 60 miles should run 36 miles the week before race week, and no more than 25 in the week before race day.

During the last four days before the marathon, don't do any runs of more than 3 miles. If you'd rather take the last two days completely off, that's OK too. Don't worry about mileage during race week – you'll get your fill on race morning.

Maintain the intensity: Even though you are cutting back on your mileage, it's important to maintain the intensity of these workouts. Run at close to marathon pace, so your body is accustomed to the effort level you will demand during the race.

Avoid the hills: Don't run any hills during race week – it helps your legs recover more quickly. It's just like with the mileage: your legs will get plenty of work on race day.

Choose your weapons: Decide in advance what clothes you will wear on race day. Pick comfortable shoes, socks, and running clothes that you've already worn on a long training run. DON'T wear anything new on marathon day, unless you want to have a graphic chafing story to tell your family about afterwards.

Gain a few – but not a lot: Since you are running less, pay close attention to your diet. It's normal to gain a few pounds as your muscles stockpile the glycogen they will need during the race, but gaining more than five pounds could make you feel heavy and sluggish. Eat a bit less than usual, with well-balanced meals, and don't start any fad diets this week.

Remember, carbo loading doesn't mean overloading. The night before the race, just eat a regular sized meal with a higher percentage of carbohydrates than usual. On race morning, eat a small portion of a bagel, banana, or oatmeal to top off your tank – but don't load your stomach to the brim. 26 miles is a long way to run with a stomach cramp.

Wake up early: If you're not accustomed to running in the morning, try a couple of morning runs, so your body gets a taste of exercising at that time of day. Marathon start times are often at 7AM or earlier – and if you've never run at that hour, it can be a bit of a shock. You might as well get it over with prior to race morning.

Eliminate extra activities: If you do any cross training activities, don't do them during race week. Don't do any unusual activities that might cause muscle soreness afterwards. This isn't the time to catch up on housework or repair projects. If you have extra time on your hands, just read a book or take a nap instead.

(We know this rule isn't popular with spouses, but we'll take the heat on this one. Tell your spouse we said so, and he or she can write us an angry e-mail instead of venting at you. After the race, however, you're on your own.)

Cut your toe nails: Do it 5 or 6 days before the race. Trust us on this one.

Be paranoid: It's fairly common for runners to get minor illnesses while tapering, so stay away from sick people. Wash your hands after touching anybody. Make like Howard Hughes for a couple of weeks, and you'll be assured of staying healthy.

Visualize success: The mental side of marathon running is extremely important. Each day during your taper, picture yourself running relaxed and strong, and having a great race. Repeating this scenario each day will build confidence in your ability to succeed.

Enjoy yourself: Yes, you should take the precautions above – but don't get so overwhelmed with worry that you forget to enjoy the experience. Think of how far you've come in your training, and resolve to have a great time on race day.

And then all that's left is to go out and do it!

Red Badge of Courage

Warning: this column contains graphic depictions of sensitive body areas. Reader discretion is advised.

Winter is rapidly approaching, which for most people means celebrating the joys of the season; ski weekends, school vacations, and nervous laughter as your boss gets hammered at the company party – things like that.

On the other hand, many runners become preoccupied by thoughts of flaming thighs, misty butt, and udder cream.

Cold weather forces runners to wear extra layers of clothing, which can irritate the skin in many places. For them, winter 'tis the season for increased chafing. So even though it may make you wince or grimace, today we're gonna talk about it. (No need to thank us. We consider this a public service.)

It's a problem as old as the sport itself. The first recorded case of chafing afflicted one of the lesser-known Knights of the Round Table, Sir Chafealot (thus the word origin). After a long day on horseback slaying enemies of the king, Sir Chafealot was heard to complain, "Forsooth and alas! My inner thighs feeleth hot as dragon's breath."

Runners definitely know how Sir Chafelot feels. Virtually all of us, at one time or another, have had what's sometimes called the Red Badge of

Courage: a particularly nasty case of chafing that grows worse with each passing mile.

Sure, you may decide to gut out the pain and finish the run – but then you end up walking bowlegged for a week and screaming bloody murder anytime you get in the shower. Every subsequent run feels like your skin is peeling off. Alas indeed.

Chafing can occur anywhere that skin rubs against skin, or against certain types of clothing. The most common areas are the inner thighs, but virtually every part of the body is fair game; the longer the run, the greater the chance of chafing.

If you don't believe us, watch the finish of a marathon someday, where you'll encounter members of the Bloody Nipple Society. When cotton shirts or other coarse fabrics rub against unprotected nipples for several hours, the results are sometimes horrific. It can happen to both men and women. Sometimes it takes weeks to completely heal.

Scarlet Cleft Syndrome is a relatively underreported medical condition caused by running in tights. Many runners wear tights or compression shorts to reduce the occurrence of inner thigh chafing. Unfortunately, if the tights are too snug at the waist, or have thick seams, they can cause this syndrome at the top of the buttocks – a mark known endearingly as "mistybutt."

You may be surprised to hear that this topic has actually been researched. Dr. Andrew McMillan from the University of Glasgow in Scotland, in a particularly enlightening study, concluded that, "Contact between buns and fabric tends to become troublesome when layering is involved." Um, no kidding.

Dr. McMillan suggests running sans underwear beneath the tights, and that for females, "thongs and g-strings can be problematic." (Remember, that's only while running. Otherwise we're very much in favor.)

So how can runners prevent excess chafing during the winter months?

Thankfully, there's an entire industry devoted to keeping runners' tender areas tender. Several chafe protection products are available; the most popular one is probably BodyGlide, a balm that comes in a deodorant-style dispenser, which can be rubbed on sensitive areas. It also has SPF for sun protection – but if you're having trouble with sunburn in your private areas, we suspect your problem might not be running-related. Similar products on the market include Runner's Lube, Chafe Eez, and Bag Balm.

Many runners swear by Udder Cream, which was designed to keep cow udders from getting chafed by milking machines. It's available in most feed stores or hardware stores. No, we're not making this up. Some resourceful (or maybe just cheap) runners use Crisco or Pam right out of their kitchen cabinets. Others use Johnson's baby oil, Desitin, Gold Bond powder, Balm X, or other bathroom remedies that you've always heard about but never really knew what they were used for.

One runner's website has an expert suggestion for mixing your own formula with various ingredients including A&D ointment, vitamin E and Aloe vera cream. Never question the lengths that runners will go to protect their valuables.

Of course, the most predominantly used product is that old-school classic, Vaseline. Many elite marathoners extol the virtues of petroleum jelly. Frank Shorter, the last American to win a gold medal in the Olympic Marathon, gave a clinic at the Big Sur Marathon expo several years ago. One runner asked Frank exactly how he prevents chafing.

Frank's answer was simple: he uses Vaseline. But apparently he felt he didn't elaborate enough, so he continued: "I use it everywhere. EVERYwhere. EVERYWHERE! I use it on my legs. I use it on my toes. I use it on my arms. Whatever place is in your mind – I use it there too. EVERYWHERE!"

Far be it from us to argue with Frank on this one – so go ahead and use Vaseline sometime. Use it everywhere.

Your choice of clothing is also very important. Better fitting clothes will reduce your chance of gaining a Red Badge. If you wear tights, make sure the seams are soft and don't lie over delicate areas. With shirts, moisture wicking fabrics are very effective at moving sweat away from your body, preventing the shirt from becoming heavy and coarse. Many runners also wear Band-Aids to decrease their risk of developing nipple "issues."

Thankfully, chafing doesn't have to be inevitable. With a little trial and error you should be able to find the right combination of products that work best for you. Once you find a system that works, stick with it.

Then hopefully you won't end up like Sir Chafealot this winter.

Get Your Drink On

When temperatures grow warmer, runners need to pay extra attention to hydration needs when exercising in the heat. In recent years, hydration devices have become very prolific, with multiple styles and options available.

As a general rule, unless you're exposed to extreme heat or humidity (upper 90s for either category), you probably don't need to take in fluids during your workout if you are exercising for 30 minutes or less. If you are exercising for less than an hour, you can probably do just fine with water instead of sports drink.

When your body is working for more than one hour, make sure that you drink small amounts of fluid on a regular basis during the activity. There are a few different ways to carry fluids on the go:

Handheld bottle carriers: Of course, before hydration accessories were invented, everybody did it the old fashioned way: by carrying a bottle of water in your hand while you run. Handheld bottle carriers are little more than a comfortable elastic strap that fits around the bottle and the back of your hand; this way, you don't have to grip the bottle to keep it in contact with your palm.

Most handheld carriers support a 20-oz bottle, and many have small pockets on the backside to stash things like keys or an ATM card. Some runners find it awkward to carry bottle holders at first, but before long you'll hardly notice a difference.

Waist Packs: These are probably the most common option, and come in several varieties. Most packs hold a 20- or 24-oz bottle on your backside, often angled one way or the other to help with quick access. Waist packs also have larger pockets with more storage space for cell phones or energy bars.

Variations on this design include packs that hold two full-size bottles, and others with several smaller bottles distributed all the way around your waist. In our opinion, the single bottle option is the simplest and most convenient, and should suffice for activity in the one to two hour range.

If you are running or hiking for more than two hours, a single bottle won't be enough to sustain you – and that's where the next category comes in.

Hydration Packs: These lightweight packs are typically worn like a backpack, but contain a fluid reservoir that can hold up to 100oz of fluid. Models that are intended for runners typically hold about 70 oz.

Since they are designed for longer activity, hydration packs also feature a lot more storage space for food, clothing, or other gear. Modern materials and designs make these packs quite comfortable to wear, even when running at high speed.

Fluid reservoirs are slightly more high-maintenance than a typical water bottle – they're a bit more difficult to clean and dry after each use – but they're generally very easy to use, and the benefit of having adequate fluids during a long run is usually worth a little inconvenience afterwards.

Handheld bottle carriers and waist packs can be found at most local running stores. If you'd like more information about hydration packs, Donald has tested and reviewed several of them for his website at www.runningandrambling.com, and an Internet search will also provide you plenty of reviews to get started.

Whichever method you choose, be sure to take care of your hydration needs so you can enjoy a healthy and safe summer of running.

Donald Buraglio and Michael Dove

Opening the Mailbag (1)

(Author's note: once our column was up and running, so to speak, we periodically received e-mails from runners with various inquiries, which we occasionally compiled into newspaper articles to share the information with everyone. Two of them appear in this book collection.)

The following are real questions from real runners ...

Should I wear headphones when I run? This is one of the most popular questions we hear. Now that portable music players are extremely small, and headphones are very durable, many people are taking their tunes along with them while working out. They find that music can be motivational, invigorating, and make the time go by quicker on longer runs.

Unfortunately, headphones can be extremely dangerous in many situations that runners commonly encounter. If you run on roads, you always have to be alert for approaching cars, and in other areas you need to be aware of cyclists and pedestrians around you. Even just running through your neighborhood, you need to react to wandering dogs or cars pulling out of driveways. In any of these situations, headphones will significantly impact your reaction time and jeopardize your safety. And hopefully it goes without saying that if you run in the dark of early mornings or late evenings, headphones are ABSOLUTELY unsafe.

Having said that, there are certain situations where headphones would be OK. If you are running laps around the outside lanes of the track, or if you are trying to block out the lame pick-up lines of that annoying guy at the health club, you have our blessing to make like Eminem and just lose yourself in the music, the moment.

Both of us prefer to be in tune with the surroundings rather than surrounded with the tunes, but your preferences may differ.

What are the best exercises for improving my running? This may surprise you, but don't focus on your legs; work on your abdomen instead. Strengthening your core region improves your running efficiency and helps prevent injury. There are many ways to strengthen your abdominal region, but the easiest way is to go "low-tech" and do basic crunches, floor exercises on a mat, or use a physioball.

Plyometric exercises - strengthening exercises that utilize a muscle's stretch reflex - are also beneficial. Many of these exercises are old-school also, incorporating various types of jumping or bounding. Get some instruction from an athletic trainer before trying these.

Consistency is the key for these activities- try to do these supplemental exercises at least twice per week.

When should I stretch? (or, should I stretch at all?) There have always been arguments about the value of stretching, but we feel it is an important component of running. Stretching cold muscles is largely ineffective, so it's better to skip the pre-run stretching and just start your first mile slowly. Stretching after a run is good to decrease short-term soreness and to maintain long-term flexibility in your muscles. It is especially important for older runners, as muscles gradually lose their natural elasticity over time. Stretch until the point where you feel a slight pull, and hold that position for about 30 seconds. You should never stretch to the point of hurting.

Won't running hurt my knees? Not if you start properly and avoid common mistakes. If you are obese or sedentary to start with, you need to begin an exercise program very gradually, and let your body adapt to the new strains placed on it. Knee pain is a typical symptom of runners who try to progress their workload too quickly. You also need to pay attention to your footwear, as this plays a role in injury prevention.

Over the long term, there have been no reliable studies showing that runners have a higher incidence of arthritis than the non-running population in general. So yes, your uncle who ran for 10 years may have arthritis now, but chances are he was destined to develop it anyway. Additionally, the health benefits of a regular running program far outweigh the risk that your knees might hurt you later on.

Should I use energy gels when running? We think energy gels like GU, Power Gel and CLIF Shot are very helpful during marathons, to prevent the dreaded "bonk" during the final miles. For recreational runners, they are largely unnecessary until you are exercising for 90 minutes or more. For any less time than that, water or a sports drink are adequate to fuel your workout. If you're training for a marathon and plan on using a gel during the race, be sure to practice using them during your long training runs as well.

Thanks again for all of your correspondence, and keep those e-mails coming!

GPS Depression

After one of our runs last week with some of our faster running partners we caught yet another case of GPS Depression. Allow us to explain, and see if you might sympathize with us.

We had just finished the usual Friday route when Dave asked, "How long was that run?"

Andrew looked at the GPS device on his wrist and said, "I've got it at 6.78 miles with 1,142 feet of elevation change."

Jim looked at his device and said "My GPS says it was 6.52 miles with 948 feet of elevation change, and our average pace was 6.43 minutes per mile."

Jon said, "*My* GPS says it was 6.84 miles with 1,045 feet of elevation change, and our average pace was 6:35 minutes per mile. Also, the average temperature was 38.6 degrees, and our speed of inertia correlation coefficient had a Beta factor of 1.23."

Dave yelled, "Hey – all I wanted was to know if we ran 45 minutes or not … I have to get to work!"

All that we got from this was another case of GPS Depression.

It started with mild confusion over the distances being different on each GPS device. Did we run 6.78 miles, which could be logged in our mileage books as six and three-quarters? Or did we actually run 6.84 files, which could be rounded up to 7? Or was the mileage officially less than six and a half?

There's an old saying that, "the man with one watch ALWAYS knows what time it is, but the man with more than one NEVER knows" – and this situation made us appreciate the wisdom of that sentiment quite profoundly.

Our day to day confusion in cases like this soon gave way to utter depression, as each week the GPS measured the distance of this regular Friday run at substantially less than we historically recorded. Until the GPS devices found their way into our running group, the Friday run was universally agreed upon as 7.5 miles; we have many years of 7.5s in our running logs to prove it.

So now we find ourselves with a dilemma – and we're sure it's one that many of you share. Could it be that many of those miles from all those runs we've been recording over the years are bogus? Do we have to go back and correct all our yearly running logs now? When we were running 50 mile weeks were they actually 48? When we felt proud about hitting 80 miles per week, was it actually more like 75? To non-runners, these seem like trivialities – but to dedicated runners, they are the makings of a nightmare.

The bad dream gets even worse – because on every one of our training runs, a similar phenomenon occurs. Our 13-mile Tuesday run is actually 12.7. Our Wednesday run is 6.4 instead of our historically recorded 7. Our one-mile time trial course is only 0.98 miles long. Our weekend 20-milers may be as short as 18. And why does the GPS *never* say a run is *longer* than we think? It's enough to make a runner seek out some antidepressants.

We can rationalize by considering the limitations of GPS devices. There are always questions about their precision, particularly on trail routes that are in narrow canyons or have a lot of tree cover. Sometimes the GPS devices lose their signals and recover by picking up again at a new location, thus missing a bit of mileage. Our egos have decided that this is certainly what must be occurring on ALL of our routes.

The irony of this story is that at many races, GPS users are known to claim that the course measures longer than the advertised distance. The Big Sur Half Marathon is an officially registered course of 13.1 miles; representatives of USA Track and Field measure the distance using state of the art calibration, and grant their official designation that the race is certified. However, after the race some GPSers always complain that their measurements were 13.2 or 13.3 miles.

The primary reason for this discrepancy is that course measurement is based on taking every tangent and short angle possible through every turn. In a crowded field of runners on a sometimes narrow road, very few runners aside from the lead pack are able to run every single one of these tangents.

The route is short, the course is long … you can never completely please a GPS wearer.

Fortunately, we found a savior in the Beta factor, which might be precisely the anti-depressant we've been looking for. After that memorable Friday run that caused so much consternation, Jon e-mailed us later to say that when he plugged his GPS watch into his computer running analysis program it confirmed the beta factor on our 6.8 mile run was 1.23.

This means that because of all the hills we ran and our average speed, our 6.8 miles could be multiplied by 1.23 to arrive at the actual training value of our run in miles. That comes out as 8.4 miles of training value. Who knew? Our 7.5 mile route was actually only 6.8 miles but then magically we were getting 8.4 miles of value from it. We love the Beta factor!

But now, do we record 6.8 miles, or 7.5 miles, or 8.4 miles with an asterisk in our log? Or should we should just record 45 minutes? We sorely miss the days when running used to be so easy.

**Postscript: about three weeks after this article appeared, Jon confessed that he made the whole Beta thing up just to mess around with us. So much for feeling good about ourselves.*

The Perfect Day

Runners hear a lot of advice; sometimes, too much advice.

Don't get us wrong – we're all for healthy living and eating. But you can drive yourself crazy trying to do everything that experts recommend.

To illustrate this point, we've gathered a large sampling of advice and put together a blueprint for a Perfectly Healthy Day. How many of these things can you claim in your daily routine?

1. Wake up early, at the same time every day – even on weekends.
2. Enjoy a few minutes of conversation with your loving spouse.
3. Get out of bed and drink your first of 8 glasses of water for the day.
4. Brush and floss your teeth – the first of three times today.
5. Eat a pre-exercise snack of a half bagel or an energy bar.
6. Do warm-up exercises while watching the news to stay intellectually current.
7. Meet the running group before dawn for your daily run of 30 to 60 minutes – longer on weekends.
8. Stay socially connected with the runners by discussing family, politics, philosophy, and sharing some laughs during the run.
9. Afterwards, do your post-run stretching and yoga. Drink more water.
10. Eat a healthy breakfast together with the family. Be sure to include whole grains, antioxidants, flaxseed oil, and lots of fiber.
11. Vitamin time! Toss down a multi-vitamin plus vitamins C and E, with a selenium or coenzyme Q10 chaser. Are you female? Don't forget the iron, calcium and vitamin D. Male? Take lycopene for prostate health. Over 40? Glucosomine

and chondroitin, ginkgo biloba, and 2 baby aspirin. Under 10? Flintstones.

12. Drink a cup of black coffee or green tea for extra antioxidants.
13. Off to work for a day of rewarding, meaningful employment that you love. Carpool to work, ride your bike, or drive in your hybrid car.
14. Listen to National Public Radio in the car – but occasionally scroll across the rap or rock stations to stay aware of what your kids are listening to.
15. Park far away from your office so you can burn extra calories walking to the door. If it's a multi-story office building, never use the elevator.
16. Do some early-morning meditation at your desk, and visualize a successful day.
17. Maintain healthy relationships with all your co-workers to decrease stress. Treat every problem as a new opportunity.
18. Have a mid-morning snack of nonfat yogurt and a few walnuts or almonds.
19. Drink another helping of water, black coffee or green tea. Then stop drinking caffeine after noon.
20. Call or e-mail your spouse and family during the day to see how they are doing (but not on company time – be sure to clock-out first). While you're at it, call your parents and touch base with your siblings. Always tell people how much you love them.
21. Lunch time! Enjoy your fruit cup or garden salad. Drink water instead of soda. Go for a short walk outside after eating.
22. Take a 20-minute power nap in the early afternoon, and then get back to work! Your co-workers are looking for you.
23. Get up from your desk and do some stretches every hour.
24. Afternoon snack: two pieces of dark chocolate (at least 70% cocoa content), along with an apple or banana.
25. Reserve 10 minutes before the end of the workday to straighten your desk and compile a "to do" list for the next day. This assures that tomorrow will be low-stress and productive.

26. Take your hybrid car, bicycle, or carpool home.
27. At least once per week, get a massage after work to release muscle tension.
28. After work, have a nice conversation with your spouse, spend some quality time with each of your kids, or do some volunteer work at your church or synagogue.
29. Before dinner, have one glass of red wine with high resveritrol content. (You'll find the highest content in Dr. Constantine Franks Pinot Noir from New York; that's our vinicultural tip of the week).
30. Eat dinner together as a family every night, no later than 6:30 PM.
31. For dinner, have a main course of salmon (wild, not farmed) at least twice per week to get your Omega 3's and 6's. Have bright, colorful vegetables along with it. On the other nights have small portions of pasta with very light sauce, plus lean meat or chicken.
32. Try to skip dessert. But if you can't resist, then have some lowfat pudding or try a dessert recipe from *Cooking Light* magazine.
33. Once you get up from the table – that's it. No more eating for the night.
34. Spend individual time with each of your children separately before bedtime. Participate in their bedtime routines.
35. Time to catch up on TV – good thing you have TiVo. Watch a one-hour show in 44 minutes. Do some sit ups or stretching while you watch. Remember to limit your TV to one hour a night, and then go read a self-help or motivational book. Or work on a Sudoku or crossword puzzle to stay mentally sharp.
36. Talk to your spouse for at least 30 minutes before bedtime.
37. Get to bed early so you can get at least 7 hours of sleep. End the day with some hugs, cuddling, and maybe (if you're lucky) some intimacy with your spouse.
38. Fall asleep easily, make all of your dreams pleasant ones.

So how did you do? Clearly, it's pretty tough to have a perfect day. If your answer is a low number, don't worry – so is ours. But that doesn't stop us from continually trying.

Opening the Mailbag (2)

Here are real questions from real runners we've received recently …

I always see runners jogging in place on street corners while they wait for the lights to change. Is there any benefit to that? Most people's reactions to seeing someone bobbing up and down on a street corner dressed in running clothes is a mixture of mockery and pity. It may surprise you to hear that we completely agree.

Let's face it, bouncing on a street corner looks pretty goofy. It's like an open invitation for drivers to scoff at the "silly runner." And there's really no training benefit from hopping up and down in the middle of a run to try to keep moving for a few extra seconds. So our advice is, just DON'T do it.

If you simply must keep moving, just walk back and forth a bit, or stretch your legs until the light turns green. Then continue along to the park, trail, or anyplace else away from intersections so you don't have to look like a dancing clown.

I'm 64. Is it too late to start a running program? It is never too late to start a walking or running program! We've had four runners in our Big Sur Marathon training program over the years who started running when they were 70 or older, and they all finished the marathon. Don't just take our word for it, though – because science backs us up on this one.

Several studies have shown that anyone can reverse many of the negative effects of poor nutritional and fitness habits if they stick to a running program for 6 months and modify their diet. In other words, even if you are a lifetime couch potato, you can still lower your blood pressure and cholesterol, decrease your chances of getting cancer or heart disease, reduce your stress levels, improve your immune system, and gain other benefits from beginning an exercise program.

So get out there, Grandma!

Should I say hello or wave to other runners as they go by? We love questions about social etiquette while running. On this subject, the answer is somewhat influenced by where you run and how many other runners you see.

Most people enjoy a smile and a hello. But if you're running in a busy area like Monterey's coastal recreation trail on a beautiful summer afternoon, and there are hundreds of walkers, joggers, inline skaters, or moms with stroller-fitness groups sharing the trail with you, you'll lose your voice trying to say hi to everybody.

In most situations, when runners are few and far between, it's usually a nice gesture to wave and acknowledge other runners as they go by. Just by being out there running, you're sharing a common experience, and probably have similar lifestyles.

There are two ways to approach the greeting:

When going in opposite directions: Go ahead and say hello or "good morning" or whatever greeting you are comfortable with. You can also do wordless acknowledgements like a smile or a slight nod, or a slight upward move of the hand and wrist that could be interpreted as a wave.

It's probably a good idea to avoid high-fives – especially if the gal coming the other way is a 64-year-old woman who is new to running. The last thing we want is to cause a rash of shoulder injuries.

When going in the same direction: This is a situation of one runner (or group) passing another, so be careful not to say anything that might be demeaning. A simple hi or good morning work well here, but you'll probably have a few extra seconds to comment on the weather or ask about a logo on someone's shirt.

Be aware, however, that some runners aren't overly chatty – so if you make a couple of charming comments and don't get a response, the other person may just prefer to run in silence. (Either that, or she's just not into you – but that's a whole separate column.)

Should I run every day or take a few days off per week? This one depends entirely on your goals as a runner and your reasons for running. Competitive national-class runners run twice a day. Most competitive age-groupers run every day. For recreational runners we suggest you run 4 or 5 days a week for 30 minutes to an hour each time.

If you get "edgy" by having a day without running or exercising, then cross-train by riding a bike, swimming, walking, or going to the gym for some strength work. Your body will thank you for the days off.

That's all we have room for today – Happy Running!

OH THE PLACES YOU'LL RUN!

"'We call it the Jesus trail,' he said with deliberate significance intended, 'and I run with Muslims and Christians and Jews. We all get along fine! If everyone was a runner we would have peace here!'"

"But here's the even greater thing: the Dipsea trail is open every day of the year. West Sands Beach is available to anybody who wants to travel there and experience it. The same is true of any of the most famous locations in running. Unlike any well-known athletic stadium, you don't have to 'know somebody' to get in. It's part of the charm of our sport."

Strawberry Fields

Occasionally I (Donald) can take some time in the middle of the day to go for a run through the fertile fields of the Salinas Valley.

The *campos* are generally laid out in a large grid pattern, with major thoroughfares paved, and the others simple dirt roads. It's a convenient place to run, because there are many opportunities to shorten or lengthen the distance as necessary, depending on how much time I have available.

The aromas of the fields vary with the seasons, and I've learned to avoid particular grids simply because of the smells I anticipate there. Certain crops have a powerfully unpleasant odor when baking in the sun all day. And needless to say, when it's time for fertilizing any of the fields, I make a beeline upwind.

Summer is the best time of year to be in the fields, as the overwhelming smell is the sweet fragrance of strawberries. One of my favorite sensory experiences in the whole world is running through the *campos* and smelling the berries with every breath I inhale.

The visual effect is also pretty cool. The tops of the bushes are covered with leaves, and as I cruise between adjacent fields, I feel like I'm sailing through a lush green ocean, with a strawberry-scented sea breeze in my face.

In the *campos*, I also witness the labor that harvests the strawberries I'm so fond of.

I see the teams of migrants who walk through the bushes bent over at the waist, gathering countless boxes that are placed in cartons alongside each row. I watch a separate group carry the cartons across the field and into a nearby truck, where another team awaits to sort and stack the berries for delivery to the produce company.

Sometimes there are as many as 100 people working the same grid, but I frequently drift past them almost unnoticed, as the entire crew remains focused on the task at hand.

Since I'm usually in the fields at midday, I run past some workers on their lunch breaks. They sit in the roads on the fringes of the fields, leaning against their cars to utilize whatever shade they can find in the summer heat. Their clothes and bodies are filthy, and they sit quietly to save their energy to get through the remainder of the day.

I know their bodies probably ache from the strain of hard labor. By comparison, the fatigue of a strenuous run is trivial.

I know that most of them will go home and share a house with many other workers, living in conditions we normally associate with third-world poverty. I know that many of them left wives and children behind to work in these conditions. I know that they sleep restlessly, worried about their health or their security or their ability to provide for their families. I know that the next morning, they'll wake up and do the same routine all over again.

In those moments, there's definitely a guilty feeling when I glide past them in expensive running shoes, wearing colorful high-performance workout clothes, peering at them from behind darkened glasses, taking a midday break from a job that pays me more in a month than they may see in half a year.

I sometimes wonder what they think when they see me. I'm sure it's some mixture of resentment and envy and disregard, but you would never tell by their expressions. When I pass in front of them and our eyes meet, I'll lift my hand and say a quick hello, and occasionally I'll get a head nod or a short greeting in reply. Then we go on with our respective tasks.

But when I finish my run and see the layers of dirt stuck to my legs from the windblown soil, I realize how much dust might be in their lungs. When I notice the tan lines from my running shorts, I remember how harmful spending day after day in the sun can be. When I feel the soreness in my legs, I consider the damage their bodies endure just to make it to the next day.

And sometimes when I smell the beautiful fragrance of strawberry fields, I think that for some people, perhaps that smell is not particularly sweet.

Running in the Holy Land

The guard tilted his head in surprise and tightened his grip on the Uzi as I (Mike) ran by. He seemed more concerned with observing the Judean hills outside the wire fence than watching me suffer in the summer desert heat. I followed the paved road hugging the inside of the fence line around the perimeter of Ofra, a settlement in the *Gush Etzion,* the West Bank. It was my first run since winning a silver medal in the half marathon at the Maccabiah Games, the Jewish Olympics, three days before.

Ofra, a settlement of mostly Americans with a pioneer spirit, is the home of my brother-in-law and his family. It is a 45-minute drive from Jerusalem. Yesterday's drive was uneventful but my wife and I were concerned when the driver commented that, "in case of trouble there are guns under the seats." He told us of rock throwing and skirmishes with Arab settlers that sounded more in spirit like fraternity pranks rather than life and death struggles.

The run was therapeutic and my mind went back to the half marathon. The rolling hills were quiet and the setting sun cast strange shadows on the road in front of me. At the ten mile mark in the race I slowly passed two other runners, one of whom tried to stay with me. He hung on about two strides behind for at least a mile before I heard him speak in Hebrew, "*Na-a-la-yeem Ya-fot.*" When I didn't react, he yelled again, "*Na-a-la-yeem Ya-fot!*" but I still didn't react. The third time he pulled up on my shoulder and waited until he had my eye contact before repeating "*Na-a-la-yeem Ya-fot!*" I shrugged my shoulders to indicate I didn't understand.

"Nice shoes!" he said in deliberate but perfect English.

"You have nice shoes!" he repeated.

I waited to talk to him after the race. He explained that running shoes were very hard to purchase in Israel and most stores carried shoe models that were at least two years behind. I questioned him on other aspects of running in Israel. How did he train in such intense heat? Was it safe? Where did he run? He explained that his favorite training run was between Jerusalem and Bethlehem because it was relatively flat.

"We call it the Jesus trail," he said with deliberate significance intended, "and I run with Muslims and Christians and Jews. We all get along fine! If everyone was a runner we would have peace here!"

As I continued my run around Ofra I considered my shoes with new meaning. I approached the top of a ridge as the sun descended toward the horizon. I glanced toward it just as it fell behind the top of a large bush that people in the United States would call tumbleweed. The bush glittered a brilliant red color from the light behind it, and it caused me to stop running and stare. I walked toward the bush with an immediate understanding about Biblical miracles. I paused and felt lucky to enjoy what I considered rare insight. At that instant I thought I heard a voice calling my name loudly in Hebrew. "*Me-Chi-Ale,*" it said, and then repeated more softly, "*Me-Chi-Ale.*"

I quickly turned in the direction of the bush, and looked in all directions, but found no one in my view.

The voice repeated my name again and then asked, "Do you want to improve your running and your life?"

"That would be wonderful," I commented.

"Then listen to me carefully and remember these ten rules that you must follow," the voice said sternly.

The voice continued, "Listen to me alone. Do not take advice from anyone else. I will be your only coach!"

"Run only for the enjoyment of running and testing yourself in competition. Don't run for the medals or glory!"

"You can tell anyone where you received this advice, but make sure you state it correctly."

I was sorry I didn't have a pen to record what I was hearing, yet somehow I remember it vividly today virtually word for word and with every intonation.

"Always take a day of rest from your training every week. Preferably on Saturday as it is before your long run on Sunday."

"Consider whether you inherited fast twitch or slow twitch muscle fiber from your mother and father and honor them by developing your training schedule accordingly."

I pondered this one and decided I needed more speedwork and interval sessions.

"But speed kills! Prepare for speed sessions with proper warm up and cool down. Don't do more than two speed sessions a week!"

"Only run hard every other day. On your rest days run very, very slowly. It is OK to run with your wife on these slow days. Don't ever run with women other than your wife!"

The sun was disappearing behind the bush and the voice spoke to me more quickly as the sky started to darken.

"Eat properly and take extra supplements of vitamins C, E and beta carotene. Do not steal snacks as you only hurt yourself!"

"Don't take a 'holier than thou' attitude about your running and your fitness. Don't preach to your friends and neighbors about your lifestyle or talk behind their backs about their bad habits."

The voice spoke very loudly and expressed each word more distinctly. "Don't be tempted by your neighbors and friends to search for short term enjoyments and pursuits. Train consistently and for the long term. Keep your goals in sight and constantly strive for them!"

I said, "Is there anything else?"

There was no response and I started to run back to my brother-in-law's house.

There was complete stillness as I resumed my pace in the Judean countryside. My mind was clear and I felt a strange calmness. After about a half mile, I saw the form of a person moving toward me in the near darkness. As we got closer I could see it was a man wearing a white robe and sandals and carrying a shepherd's staff. I was surprised that he also was running. He moved very smoothly with a marathoner's gait, his sandals barely rising above the ground with each stride and his robe flowing behind him. I could see the perspiration glistening in his mustache and beard as he shuffled by.

As we passed, he smiled and whispered, "*Shalom* - peace be with you."

Racing Away

At various times in our running careers, each of us has enjoyed participating in marathons around the country, and we've learned that there are a lot of considerations for racing away. We've also had our share of problems, so we've compiled a list of tips to help you avoid our mistakes and have a successful experience the next time you're traveling for a big race.

SAVE YOUR SIGHTSEEING FOR AFTER THE RACE. This one seems obvious, but it's difficult to just sit in your room waiting and resting when you're in New York City, Washington D.C., or any metropolitan area with lots of attractions. It's tempting to arrive several days early and schedule yourself some tours, but trust us - don't do it.

The best time to arrive is two days prior to your race. Go to the expo the next day to get your race number, but don't do much else. Schedule your tourist visits and fine dining for the days after the race; by that time, walking around the city streets will actually help your muscle recovery.

ADJUST TO TIME CHANGES BEFORE YOU GO. You can start correcting for jet lag before your departure by getting up a slightly earlier each day until your body is nearly on eastern or central time on the day you leave. This is a relatively simple strategy that really works to maintain your energy level when leaving the West Coast.

KNOW THE COURSE BEFORE YOU GO. The websites of virtually all major races have course profiles showing elevation changes, so you can familiarize yourself with the locations of all the hills on the course. Knowing the course will help you determine how hard to press the early pace, and how much energy to save for the hills awaiting you down the road.

DON'T ASSUME YOU'LL FIND YOUR FAVORITE FOOD. Even though you may be heading to a big city, don't count on finding your special pre-race meal in the local supermarket. If there's any food that you absolutely need to have with you before or during the race, pack it with you so you're not scrambling around the city trying to find it. If you drink coffee before races, don't forget to pack your favorite blend with you as well.

TAKE THE ELITE BUS OR VAN FROM THE AIRPORT. This one is a bit tricky, but some big-city marathons have booths or special VIP representatives set up in the baggage claim area of the airport. Race representatives are usually waiting to take elite runners from the airport to their hotels in vans or SUVs – and often, these vans have many extra seats.

Have a little *chutzpah* and ask the people at the booth when they are headed into town. With a bit of luck there will be extra seats and you'll save big bucks in taxi fees. The volunteers who are there are usually bored anyway from waiting and are more than willing to make you happy for the cost of a fair tip.

CHECK THE WEATHER. This might be obvious as well, but be sure to check online for the race weekend forecast and pack accordingly. In 2007, the Chicago Marathon and Twin Cities Marathons saw temperatures close to 90 degrees with very high humidity in early October, which took many participants by surprise.

Spring and fall race temperatures can fluctuate wildly in any area of the country, but you can usually get an idea of what kind of conditions you'll be in for on race day before you leave home, and pack accordingly.

CHECK YOUR HOTEL LOCATION. There are often a lot of cancellations close to marathon day and you possibly can upgrade your hotel location at the last minute.

But the key question is – what is a location upgrade? It depends on the race course. If the start and finish areas are the same, the decision is easy: stay as close to it as possible. You'll be able to sleep in later, then roll out of bed and walk to the starting line. After the race, you have a very short distance to cover before taking a nap back in your room.

If the marathon is a point to point course, arrangements can be more difficult. Find out ahead of time whether there are buses to the start line or from the finish area, and decide which area will be a more convenient location to stay.

Typically the race headquarters hotel is the most convenient for most runners' needs; our recommendation is that it's usually worth spending a few extra bucks to stay there if you can, or very close to it if that hotel is already full.

STAYING WITH FRIENDS CAN BE RISKY. Of course you might opt to stay with friends you know in the race city, but this can be problematic as well. Just because it's in the same town doesn't automatically mean that your buddy's house is convenient to where you want to be. And if your pal's not a runner, he might not understand that nachos, margaritas, and late night conversation aren't the ideal recipe for the night before a race. Sleep in the hotel on race night, and meet your friend for the fiesta afterward.

Wherever you may be running away to for your goal race, just follow our advice and you'll do fine. We wish you great weather and a personal best day!

Donald Buraglio and Michael Dove

Running Through History

The running life often leads us to exciting, historic places.

Most mainstream sports have landmark venues that are nearly sacred to their devoted fans.

The trouble is, everyday fans never get to experience what it would be like to compete in those hallowed arenas. Runners, on the other hand, get to visit the most famous locations in their sport anytime they wish.

Think of how cool it would be to play a touch football game at Lambeau Field, take batting practice at Yankee Stadium, or play a pickup game of hoops in Pauley Pavilion at UCLA. That's exactly what runners can experience when traveling to our sport's famous landmarks. Recently both of us have run in two of the most historic and beautiful locations in the world of running. Mike traveled halfway around the world, while Donald took a short drive up the California coast.

Mike was in St. Andrews, Scotland, to play golf at the birthplace of the sport. It's common knowledge that golf has been played continuously on the Old Course for almost 500 years. However, most people – even many avid runners – aren't aware of this location's connection with running. St. Andrews is also the home of the most famous running scene ever filmed: the opening title sequence from the Academy Award-winning movie *Chariots of Fire*, filmed at West Sands Beach.

Runners and non-runners alike have been inspired by this wonderful image for 25 years. Set against Vangelis' magical theme song, several young men dressed simply in white are running on the beach. They are competitive runners, getting progressively faster as the scene continues. They are the epitome of joyful running; inspired youth in their prime.

The scene ends when they hop over a small white fence. This fence borders the first fairway at the St. Andrews Old Course.

Vangelis' theme has become a staple for many marathons and other endurance events. You can hear it virtually the entire first mile of the

Boston Marathon, and Donald heard it last summer on the slopes of Pikes Peak during the final miles of that arduous marathon.

West Sands at St. Andrews is absolutely perfect for running; very flat, with hard-packed sand more than 400 yards wide, traveling almost 2 miles from the town of St. Andrews to where the River Eden hits St. Andrews Bay. Many runners use it even in the worst of weather, as Mike experienced firsthand.

He went for a run one early morning when the wind was blowing, as it does most mornings, about 40 miles per hour. The sand drifted strongly from left to right, making it difficult to run. During the run, Mike passed another runner who used characteristically Scottish understatement in commenting, "A bit drafty, what?"

It's impossible to run on West Sands without humming the *Chariots of Fire* theme and thinking of the young men preparing for the 1924 Olympics, whose hard work and sacrifice made a great Hollywood story. In one famous scene, a coach describes runner Eric Liddell, commenting, "He's a gut runner... he digs deep." It's easy to put yourself in their shoes when running this famous stretch of coastline.

Meanwhile, much closer to home, Donald also found himself "digging deep" when he took part in the Dipsea Race last week.

The Dipsea is truly a legendary race, held in almost religious regard amongst Bay Area trail runners. It is the second oldest footrace in the country (behind only the Boston Marathon), and this June marked the 96th running from Mill Valley to Stinson Beach.

The race is one of the most rugged, as well as most accident-prone, footraces that you'll ever see. Runners finish the Dipsea Race muddy, bloody, and limping – but extremely satisfied. They know they've helped write another chapter in one of America's most storied races. For all of its difficulty, runners always look forward to having a memorable experience there.

But here's the even greater thing: the Dipsea trail is open every day of the year. West Sands Beach is available to anybody who wants to travel there and experience it. The same is true of any of the most famous locations in running. Unlike any well-known athletic stadium, you don't have to "know somebody" to get in. It's part of the charm of our sport.

Runners in different cities can lace up their shoes anytime and run the course of the Boston Marathon, the New York Marathon, or San Francisco's famous (and famously crazy) Bay to Breakers. And while we wouldn't recommend it for safety reasons, Monterey County runners can run the Big Sur Marathon course on Highway 1 any day they choose.

All in all, it makes for a great way for runners to travel, whether it's across the state or around the world.

Monument Run

Whenever I (Donald) travel on business, I like to lace up my running shoes and explore the city on foot during an evening run. Running always helps me become more familiar with my surroundings – but sometimes, it teaches me larger lessons about things I'm grateful for.

Those runs are the special ones. Last month, I enjoyed just such an evening in our nation's capital.

My business day ended at 5:00 PM, leaving about 90 minutes of sunlight before night descended upon the city. I quickly changed clothes, laced up my shoes, and headed out the door of my Georgetown hotel.

I took pedestrian pathways towards downtown and noticed that several tourist groups were still making their rounds in large buses which stopped at the major monuments. I decided to use my evening run for the same purpose.

My first stop was the Jefferson Memorial at the Tidal Basin. Approaching the structure, my first realization was how large these memorials really are. Everyone knows what Washington, D.C.'s landmarks look like from photographs, but until you're standing at the base of one, it's hard to fathom their imposing size.

I ran up the marble steps and into the portico to gaze upon the 20' statue of our third President. From such a vantage point, reading his inscribed words on the walls and in the dome overhead strikes a profoundly noble chord.

I started this run seeking inspiration; less than 20 minutes in, I had found it.

My path led me around the basin to the FDR Memorial, and I slowed to walk through the waterfalls and reflecting pools. Contemplating scenes from the Great Depression, I felt thankful for the comforts I've known for my whole life.

One reason for that prosperity was the next stop on my tour: the World War II Memorial. On the west side of the plaza I stood at the Freedom Wall, taking the measure of over 4000 gold stars – each one representing 100 American deaths. Nearly all of them died younger than I am now. The evening run had taken a profoundly somber turn.

I resumed jogging along the reflecting pool toward the Lincoln Memorial. Again I was impressed by the sheer size of the monument (and I could be wrong, but it sure seemed like the steps got steeper towards the top) and the stature of the man it honors.

Despite the crowds at the base of Lincoln's chair, I noted that it was unusually silent here in the inner chamber. I could hear my own breathing as we stood in reverence of one of our country's greatest leaders.

Eventually I descended the steps and drifted over to the Vietnam Veterans Memorial. The black granite wall is simultaneously stark and sacred, and its aesthetic power was enough to stop me in my tracks.

Architect Maya Lin intended this to be a place of reflection. The granite is polished and glossy, reflecting the grass and trees and visitors that surround it. Images of life are reflected in the names of those who died, eternally connecting scenes from the present to the heroes of our troubled past.

Above all, this was a place of great sorrow, and it seemed fitting that darkness was now falling. I slowly walked the length of the wall, and then continued my journey, with just one stop remaining on my list.

I ran through Constitution Gardens toward the city's most recognizable structure. Approaching it, I saw that the lights of the Washington Monument had already been turned on, giving the towering obelisk a dusky hue against the orange and purple autumn sunset.

I ran up the sloping grass to the tower, and stood right against the monument, so the lights from the ground projected my silhouette upward against the white marble and sandstone. Standing at the base, it's impossible to see the top of the monument. Even my larger-than-life image projected up only a fraction of the tower's 555' height. The inherent message was simple: standing here, I was in the shadow of a giant.

Returning along the Potomac through the darkness, I considered the time I had just spent at these memorials. In particular, I thought of some signs I had seen along the way.

Many of the monuments have standard-issue "Quiet please – No smoking – No pets – No skateboarding" signs posted in common areas. But I was surprised to see that several of these signs also say "No running."

Was it a liability issue? Or had I somehow been disrespectful by showing up at these memorials with shorts, muddy running shoes and a sweaty Big Sur Marathon shirt? If so, I couldn't really make sense of it.

Because whether they commemorate triumphs or sadness, the monuments in our nation's capital inspire and challenge us. They force us to consider our own lives, our purposes, and how we influence the world around us.

In that regard, I thought it quite appropriate that I visited them in the midst of a run.

When I'm running, I'm filled with inspiration and encouragement. I'm never more introspective, humble, or contemplative than when I'm wearing shorts and running shoes. That night in D.C., I was especially appreciative for my abilities, and for the freedom to do the activities I enjoy.

Running in the footsteps of giants, I was also grateful to all of those who made it possible: the forefathers who made our country great, and the generations who have defended the ideals we hold dear. Sharing my run with thoughts of them is the best way I can think of to pay my respects.

And if I'm a little bit stinky and sweaty while doing so – well, hopefully Abe, George, and the others will understand.

Lessons From Spring Break

Our wives gave us a weekend pass this month to take an early Spring Break, so we didn't hesitate to load up the car and hook up with some friends for a wild road trip.

The car CD player alternated between Donald's Foo Fighters and Mike's Sugarland, but we had a like-minded purpose. We were looking for a good time with loud music, lots of drinking, fast women, and partying with thousands of people – and we knew exactly where to find it.

When we arrived in the town on Saturday, almost every motel and hotel room had been booked. All of them were filled with partygoers packed 4 to a room, just like us. Although it was a bit cold, most of the women were wearing shorts. Virtually everyone was carrying a bottle around and drinking constantly; a filmmaker could have made a video of the whole scene called "Herald Columnists Gone Wild!"

Were we in Daytona Beach or Cabo San Lucas? Sadly, no; we were in Napa, CA for the 28th annual Napa Valley Marathon. The fast-moving women in shorts were runners. Everyone's bottles were filled with water or Gatorade. We were packed 4 to a room because we're all cheap.

The Napa Valley Marathon is known for scenic vineyards and country beauty. It runs along the Silverado Trail from Calistoga to Napa, and is only trumped by Big Sur for its natural beauty and small-town charm. It's one of our favorite races.

Just to establish one point right off the bat: we're both maniacs when it comes to running. Sometimes we like running in one marathon as preparation for another. You don't have to be like us. But if you're an experienced marathoner with an ambitious time goal in an upcoming race, a "training" marathon can be very beneficial if done properly.

The key to marathon training is a weekly long run of increasing distance as you get closer to your goal race. But any runner can tell you that these runs can often become physically and mentally draining.

On the other hand, if one of your training runs has 2,000 other people, cheering spectators, and volunteers giving you Gatorade and GU every few miles, that livens things up quite a bit. And sometimes the competitive aspect helps you run a bit faster than you would on your own.

For us, our target race is usually the Big Sur Marathon at the end of April, so we use Napa Valley in early March as a long training run. There are eight weeks between races, and this is usually plenty of time to recover and gain strength again – but only if the "training" marathon is run properly.

Running a marathon is problematic on the best of days. Racing two in two months is a bit of a gamble, and experienced runners have to remember the classic advice of Kenny Rogers to deal with unpredictable race day conditions. Spring break in Napa reinforced the lessons of The Gambler. So pay attention to the following tips – because if you want to play the game, boy, you gotta learn to play it right.

Know when to hold 'em: Marathoners can never afford to get overly excited, and that's especially true in a training race. Holding a steady pace is always the best strategy. Start conservatively, and don't get carried away by the initial adrenaline rush. Usually the runners who are overly excited in the beginning are the same ones running out of gas later.

Know when to fold 'em: Everyone makes pre-race plans, or has a goal for a specific time. Unfortunately, things don't always go the way we anticipate. On race morning in Napa we faced heavy rains, cold temperatures, and sustained 30-mph headwinds. You have to be willing to throw your initial goals out the window, and revise them as necessary based on the conditions.

Know when to walk away: Sometimes your best move is to throw in your cards. At Napa Valley, Mike was nursing a sore calf muscle, and decided to stop midway through the race, rather than risk an injury that would jeopardize being healthy for Big Sur the following month.

Know when to run: Donald had the opposite experience, and felt good on race day. He recognized that he was capable of running strong despite the poor conditions, and kept a consistent pace for a very respectable 3:02 finish – which was almost exactly his target time.

Our friend and motel roommate Jim also felt great and ran an amazing 2:44 to finish 7th overall. Jim had no idea how fast he would run that day, but once he realized he was holding the aces, he turned in a fantastic race.

Never count your money when you're sitting at the table: Jim was the fastest masters (over 40) runner, and won his weight in Napa Valley wine as an award. He had no idea that he won until after he had driven home to Salinas. He's not exactly someone who is obsessed with awards.

There'll be time enough for counting when the dealing's done: Jim weighs a un-marathoner like 175 pounds, which is an awful lot of wine; we imagine he will be hosting quite a post-race celebration party.

Those were the primary lessons we brought home from Napa. As for anything else that may have transpired in those cramped hotel rooms… let's just say that what happens in Napa, stays in Napa!

Evermore

On January 1, 1975, 23-year-old Robert "the Raven" Kraft ran 8 miles in the sand on Miami's South Beach. He started running because he felt frustrated that his songwriting career was at low ebb; one of his songs had been stolen and made into a fairly large country hit and he received no credit.

A funny thing happened on that run; something that happens to a lot of people when they start running. Robert Kraft felt envigorated yet calm. His anger had mellowed, and he felt great satisfaction from those 8 miles. Like a spiritual awakening, running often finds you when you most need it.

He made running a habit. Many would call it an obsession. In fact, the Raven just completed his 34th year of running on South Beach without missing a day – a streak of more than 12,400 days in a row.

Along the way, he's become a bit of a celebrity. He is an icon on Miami Beach, and his fan base extends around the world. People travel from far and wide to run with the Raven. He maintains a list of them – one that now approaches 800 runners, from every state and 54 foreign countries. The Raven passed the 100,000 mile mark on March 29, 2009. When he did, ESPN was there to cover it.

In a sport where injuries are the norm, the Raven never misses a day to sickness or muscle pain. He runs through all kinds of weather: hurricanes, hail storms, heat and humidity. He's as reliable as the US Postal Service.

He came close to missing a run once, when he was hospitalized for a concussion and needed 17 stitches to close a nasty wound. Luckily, some lifeguard friends smuggled him out of the hospital for his daily run, then returned him after the eight miles were finished.

As you can imagine, Robert Kraft is a creature of habit. He's called the Raven because he always wears black spandex shorts, black socks, a black headband, and one wide black wristband. He has long black hair, mustache, and beard. He always runs shirtless and has a dark tan.

The Raven's also a bit of a philosopher. He chose 8 miles for his run because, "7 miles seems too short, and 9 seems too long." He runs the same 8 miles each day, in loops starting from the 6th Street lifeguard pier. Sometimes he loops in one direction, sometimes the other. He never travels out of Miami - in fact, he doesn't even own a car.

The Raven never does races. He runs for the simple pleasure of how it makes him feel, although he admits that his streak has become an obsession.

Nicknames are a big part of his persona, as Mike and his family found out while running with the Raven during a vacation to South Beach. During the run, the Raven asks you about your life, and anoints you with a nickname after you have completed the run. Then he inscribes you on "the list."

The day Mike ran there were a dozen runners who earned the nicknames Burke's Law, Chapter 11, The Reverend, Seaside Sparrow, Interrogator, Cooker, Tax Man, Wine Taster, and Unruly Julie. Mike is now known as Just Run, his wife is the Fiction Reader, his son Bryan is Pedicab Man, and Bryan's fiancée Melanie is Zot.

It is a pleasure and an honor to run with the Raven. Next time you don't feel like running, try to think like the Raven and get yourself out the door. We wish that all of us, and the Raven in particular, will continue to run evermore.

Dimensions of Compatibility

If we may ask a personal question … have you found your perfect partner in life? Someone who completes you - the yin to your yang, the cheese to your macaroni – and makes you whole? Or are you still seeking that special someone to share your future with?

In either case, this column is for you. Maybe you're currently involved with someone, but still holding out hope that a Prince (or Princess) Charming will come and sweep you off your feet. Maybe you think you're happy, but you wouldn't know any better because you've never tried anybody else, and you don't really know what the criteria would be for making a long-term commitment anyway. Maybe you don't even know what you're looking for to begin with.

Don't laugh when we say this, but picking a running partner is nearly as important to your overall wellbeing as picking a spouse. (Well, maybe you can laugh a little bit.) Accordingly, we've developed a runner's "eHarmony" test to rate your potential running mates.

For the sake of brevity, we'll assume that you can handle the logistics of meeting times and locations. The rest of the profile gets more subjective, and that's where the rating system comes into play. So get out your scorecard, and let's get started!

Timeliness: Is your partner always a few minutes early for the meeting time? Score 10. Always on time, score 5. Always late, score 0. Unpredictable - sometimes early, sometimes late - minus 5.

Pace: The best partners help you become a better runner. If your partner's comfortable pace is slightly faster than yours, score 10. Same pace, score 5. Slightly slower, score 0. Significantly slower, minus 5.

Versatility: Give your partner 5 points for each type of running terrain they enjoy: Roads. Trails. Track. Adjacent treadmills. 20 possible points.

Attitude: If your partner has a positive and enthusiastic demeanor, score 10. If it seems like he (or she) is just logging the mileage, score 5. If he frequently talks about his injuries, score 0. If he's a constant whiner, complainer, and a downer, minus 5.

Reliability: Will your partner show up when the weather is nasty? For a partner who's never intimidated by foul weather, score 10. For someone who takes on anything short of a hail storm or typhoon, score 5. For one who says he'll show up only if it's not raining, score 0. If he bails whenever there's a 30% chance of rain, minus 5.

Low maintenance: If your partner knows all the roads and trails in the area, and always comes prepared with the right gear, score 10. If he knows where to show up to meet the group every morning, score 5. If he always asks for toilet paper or a sip of your Gatorade, score 0. If he calls you late every evening to ask you what's going on tomorrow, minus 5.

Sense of humor: If your partner brings new jokes and laughs at yours, score 10. If he tells the same funny jokes a lot, score 5. If he tells jokes that aren't funny, score 0. If he tells the same unfunny jokes a lot, minus 5.

Worldly: Does he or she watch the news and know about current events? Score 10. If he likes to discuss other topics besides running, score 5. If ALL he talks about is running, score 0. If he's overbearingly political, religious, or dogmatic, minus 5.

Running Life fans: If they mention a Running Life column during a run, score 10. If they know we write a running column, score 5. If they've never heard of Buraglio or Dove, score 0. If they've written a nasty letter to the editor about us, minus 5.

OK, maybe that last category was self serving ... but it's time for the results! Check your compatibility score and place it in one of the following groups:

80 to 100: As good as it gets. Let's grow old together.

65 to 79: I'm mostly happy, but it feels like I'm settling.

50 to 64: This is OK for now, but I'd still like to see other people.

40 to 49: We need to talk. This isn't working out.

Under 40: Have a nice life. Maybe you should get a dog.

Best wishes to everyone in seeking the ideal running partner!

Donald Buraglio and Michael Dove

Runner Watching

Most runners become amazingly adept at recognizing their friends from a long distance away by their unique running styles. Even in the dark, a distinctive bounce or arm swing or posture or tilt of the head gives everyone away. Running styles become your own personal signature, almost like a fingerprint.

Some runners are regal and elegant. Some runners are blue collar and industrious. Some are prancers. Some are Clydesdales. Just head out to the local running trails or watch them as you drive by in your car and you'll see all styles and types.

One of the great things about running is that any form is acceptable. It isn't like figure skating or diving where style points count. But while some styles are OK for recreational and fitness running, the more efficient ones are definitely better for the competitive racer.

Running style is largely influenced by body type and individual biomechanics. Virtually everyone has some quirk created by leg length differences, back and abdominal strength, muscle imbalances, foot and bone structure, or other asymmetries or abnormalities that cause deviations from the ideal model.

However, running style is also dictated by personality type – and today, we're going to help you play a little game and maybe invent a new hobby. It's similar to bird watching; the object is to spot as many of these running species you can find. Or you can use this list to determine where you or your friends fit in. Here's your Runner Watching field guide.

The High Kneed Wogger: This species is identified by a very slow gait that makes it difficult to tell if the body is walking or actually running. Movement is very, very slow but definitely not a walk. The key identifying characteristic is if the knees seem to be raising vertically each step more than a walker would generally attempt.

The Type-A Burden Bearing Beast: This strange bird insists on trying to do two workouts at the same time. They can be identified because they are running while carrying weights on their arms or strapped to their legs. This Type-A insists on both ruining the joy and freedom of the running experience, while at the same time lessening the effectiveness of their strength work.

The Wing Flapping Vulture: This runner is easily identified by aggressive behavior and flapping arms. Often found running very fast with arms rotating in strange directions, this style often comes with head bobbing as well. Running close to this person can be dangerous as well as embarrassing.

The Prancing Peacock: This is typically a female of the species - does that make her a peahen? - who dresses to impress and strut her stuff. Easily identifiable by colorful clothes, this chickadee is often seen with colorful tights or running shorts accompanied by skimpy tops. This female is typically "available" and searching for a mate. Sometimes there is writing on her tail region such as "Pink" or the Greek letters of her sorority. Occasionally one can see Abercrombie on one bun and Fitch on the other.

The Bare Chested Bird of Prey: Easily identifiable on the trails by a shirtless appearance even on cold days. Typically the male of the species dresses down to impress and strut his stuff; he's obnoxious and typically "available" and searching for a mate. He sometimes flexes his muscles when running near prancing peacock, for whom he has a particular affinity. His call is typically, "How you doin', Hon?"

The Cowering Crow: Unfortunately you see this depressing runner all the time. They frown. They groan. They sneer. They grunt. They look like they would rather be doing anything but running. Typically they are fitness or weight loss runners who really don't enjoy running, but are just going through the motions because they know they should. When non-runners see this species while driving down the street, they often smile and say, "Now THAT's why I'm not a runner!"

The Happy Hummingbird: Characterized by short choppy steps and boundless energy, this runner moves from tree to bush with boundless optimism and bounce. They are a joy to watch. Try following one of these hummingbirds and you naturally try to adapt to their style and movement.

You no longer feel like running in a straight line, but suspiciously zigzag along the trail.

The Delirious Dodo: You see this runner avoiding the safer trails and running paths in favor of routes through crowded traffic areas. They run in the same direction as cars and often in the bike lanes. In the darkness they wear no reflective gear and like to wear dark colors. It is no wonder that natural selection has made them an endangered species.

The Red Breasted Novice: We have mentioned this sorry creature in other columns. They're easy to spot late in a marathon or half marathon by their distinctive red spots on the breast, caused by blood from chafed nipples without protection. The Red Breaster is sometimes not aware of the issue until after the race when he looks at his shirt in surprise and disgust. Others become aware of their red breasted status much earlier in the race because of the intense pain, and have a call that sounds like the whippoorwill, which they repeat continuously the last few miles of their race.

The Soaring Golden Eagle: The most magnificent of the species. They look like they were born to run. They move elegantly and magnificently with perfect posture. Their speed is effortless. They glide over the ground and look like they could run forever. They are often spotted at the front of large groupings of fellow runners.

Like you would with an aviary guide, we advise you to keep this column with you in your car or by your bay window, and check off the various species as they wander by. Better yet, go out into the field yourself by heading out for a run and marveling at the magnificent diversity found within the running kingdom.

Jokes on the Run

Everyone knows about the healing power of laughter – but did you know that it can also make you a better runner?

Nothing makes a run seem shorter and easier than someone sharing a great joke along the way. The longer the joke takes to tell – and the more mileage it helps to preoccupy – the better. Whenever someone tells a "shaggy dog story," the pace of the group inevitably picks up, adrenaline surges, smiles appear, and fatigue dissipates. Whether you are the storyteller or the listener, the effect is the same.

That's why it's wonderful to have someone in your running group who stays up to date on the latest jokes. It's also a great idea to have a "joke day" run when everyone in the group is required to bring a new one to share. Include some stakes to make it interesting: the worst joke teller has to buy beer or coffee after the run.

We'll get you started: There once was a running club that valued humor so much that they issued every member a copy of "The World's Best Joke Book." Each joke was numbered and everyone memorized the book. That way, instead of telling the whole joke, a runner could just yell, "Number 23!" and everyone exploded in wild laughter.

One day a new runner joined them, and tried to embrace the joke tradition by yelling, "Number 71!" There was a long, dead awkward silence and the pace slowed dramatically. Finally one of the group members said, "Nah ... you didn't tell it right!"

Obviously, this kind of group misses the point of utilizing jokes on the run. The benefit is in the telling. It's in the anticipation and mystery of the punch line. It makes time go faster. It gives camaraderie to the group.

As longtime runners, the two of us have more than a few all-time favorite jokes that are told in our group over and over again. When somebody new joins in, it won't be long before he (or she) hears all of the group favorites. And his reactions to the jokes are closely observed – sometimes, the amount of laughter will even indicate whether he is invited back to the next run. Have we mentioned yet that we take joke-telling seriously?

We'd love to share our favorite jokes here, but they would take way more column space than this skinny sidebar allows us. Besides, we're told that this is a family-oriented newspaper, and many of our jokes would definitely screw that up.

So what we'll do instead is to give you our favorite punch lines. See if you can fill in the "the rest of the story."

This might even be a fun game: can you identify any of these jokes just by their conclusions? Here are the top 10 punch lines that have entertained our running group through countless miles:

1. Somebody stole our tent!
2. Just you and me!
3. Death … by BONGO!
4. I hate playing golf with your Dad.
5. Oh, look – he's moving!
6. The chicken is a ventriloquist.
7. I don't know … it all happened so fast.
8. European!
9. What? They gave me a Chihuahua?
10. Thanks! Most people leave me on the swing.

If by chance you recognize any of them, we give you complete permission to use these jokes to improve your next run.

When the Runners and Bikers Meet

"BIKERS UP! RUNNERS UP!" If you hear this warning on a Saturday morning in Pebble Beach, pay close attention: you may soon witness an exciting and potentially dangerous encounter between two rival gangs of local endurance athletes.

Cyclists and runners are the Monterey Peninsula's version of the West Coast - East Coast rap rivalry. Both groups are enormously talented, but each one feels disrespected by the other. It's like the Sharks and the Jets from *West Side Story*: we occupy the same turf, we have a hard time seeing the other group's point of view, and we occasionally get into skirmishes. One such encounter typically happens during each group's Saturday morning workout, at a predictable time and location; so consistently you could probably set your watch to it.

Remember the old word problems from high school math? Group A, consisting of about 60 bikers, starts in Monterey at 7AM, heading south into Pebble Beach on 17-Mile Drive going 20 miles per hour. Group B contains 40 runners, starts from Carmel at 7:15 AM, and heads north into Pebble Beach at 8 miles per hour. The question is: where do these two groups meet, and at what time?

The answer is, on 17-Mile Drive about one half mile south of Bird Rock at approximately 8:00 AM. But there's much more to the story. Allow us to set the scene a bit.

The runners park in Carmel, chat a bit, and then slip on their $100 Asics or New Balance shoes they purchase 3 to 5 times per year. They wear technical fabric clothing from Sugoi or Nike, along with $200 heart rate monitors or $300 GPS units, and start as a pack. The usual run is 12 miles; 6 miles out to Bird Rock and then back. The crowd gradually strings out into several smaller, similarly-paced groups. By the time the first runners reach the turnaround, there can be as much as two miles between them and the stragglers. Conversation is rampant, but rarely about running; the most common topics are family, work, sports, or politics.

The bikers park in Monterey, chat a bit, and then start out slowly on their $2,000 to $7,000 bikes they purchase every 3 to 5 years with names like Colnago, Pinarello, or Trek. They wear $200 Sidi or DMT shoes, and are decked out in bright colors like Cirque De Soleil performers in Castelli, Pearl Izumi, or Santini duds. The usual ride is 40 miles, and when the riders hit 17-Mile drive, the hammer is dropped, with the peloton breaking into 2 main groups and a handful of stragglers. The conversations early in the ride are usually about tires, bars and stems, and components. These discussions taper off in Pebble Beach as the riders concentrate on staying in a tightly-packed group while traveling at high speeds.

So what exactly happens just south of Bird Rock? The situation is inherently problematic. Bicycle safety dictates that riders travel with traffic, on the right side of the road. Runner safety requires them to run facing traffic, on the left. Consequently, both groups are careening toward each other on the ocean side of the road. Now consider that the road has almost no shoulder, many curves and hills, and is frequently foggy, and you get a sense of the potential danger involved.

The hammering, fast moving, traveling circus of bikers pushes hard and hugs the corners. The experienced regulars start yelling, "RUNNERS UP!" even when runners are not in sight. The lead pack of runners, wanting to keep their footing on the asphalt, usually moves to the right side of the road, crossing the path of the oncoming cyclists. The experienced runners yell, "BIKERS UP!" even when bikers are not in sight. The two groups finally converge, with the bikers yelling, "D**N RUNNERS!" as they whoosh by, and the runners yelling "D**N BIKERS!" as they glide along. When the meeting is choreographed properly, injury and accidents are narrowly avoided for another week.

Unfortunately, a couple of times per year the weekly meeting results in injury, and it's almost always the biker who gets the worst of it. Runners can usually bail off the road one at a time, and they have the nearby ice plant to cushion their fall. When one biker goes down, he frequently takes the whole group with him in a heap of metal and blood and shredded Italian sportswear. It's an ugly scene that nobody likes to see. Thankfully, the rivalry hasn't quite reached Biggie vs. Tupac proportions; as far as we know, nobody has yet died in one of these altercations. And there aren't any of us who ever wish injury upon the other group.

The bikers respect the runners and the runners respect the bikers. Both groups have a passion for their chosen activity. A lot of us have shared experiences in each sport. Many cyclists are former runners (we runners call this "turning to the dark side") who find the non-impact cycling motion much easier on their joints. Many runners are former cyclists who got frustrated dealing with the equipment aspects of cycling - having to stay current with the latest gear, or getting dropped by another rider because he has the better ride. Some of us are triathletes who spend time in both camps, and understand the perspective of each side.

To the runners: understand that it's very difficult for cyclists to stay in a close pack while traveling at high speeds on a dangerous road. Please make every effort to get out of the way. To the bikers: we'll try to avoid you, but traffic conditions may not allow us to give you a whole lane of the road. Please use extra caution when riding past a long string of runners. Hopefully we can continue to share the roads without a major incident.

Just remember: BIKERS UP! RUNNERS UP!

Vacation Running

Getting away from it all doesn't require you to leave your fitness behind as well. We both find that vacation running can be an enormous pleasure with new paths, new scenery, new adventures, and new places to explore.

Often, the best way to get a feeling for an unfamiliar area is to run through its streets or trails. If you're headed out on vacation soon, here are some tips that have come in handy for us over the years:

Do advance planning: Check an online weather forecast for your destination, so you know what to pack. Different parts of the country (or beyond) could have dramatically different conditions than you're accustomed to.

Expand your web search to include running routes or clubs you can find on the road. A Google search can frequently find contact information for clubs and group runs in the area. *Runner's World* magazine also has information on its website about many national and international destinations.

Do advance reconnaissance on your lodging as well. Check if your hotel has a fitness room or treadmill for those days where you just can't get outside. Call the concierge to ask about the area surrounding the hotel. How close is it to parks, running trails, bike paths? However, take this advice with a grain of salt, as we'll explain later.

Pack sparingly: Honestly, it is much easier to run while on vacation than to play golf or tennis or ski. All you need are your shoes, socks, shirts, and shorts, as well as a watch and maybe a cap. You don't even need new clothes for every day of running – it's easy to alternate two pairs of shorts or shirts if you set them out to dry after each run. Sure, they'll smell a bit, but don't worry about it – these people don't know you, and they'll probably just think you're European.

Find a resource: When you get to town, call or visit the local running store in the area. Ask about interesting places to run, as well as upcoming group runs or special events. A local store can also advise you about areas in town to avoid in the interest of safety.

Look for an oval: Sometimes a great workout is as close as the nearest high school or college track. If you don't have time for a scheduled 2-hour run, you can maintain your fitness level by doing short-duration speed work on the track. Tracks are great places to find other runners as well; it's a runner's version of the neighborhood watering hole, only without all the drunks.

Beware the concierge: We know, we just recommended using the concierge. However, we've also run into some difficulty after taking advice from desk clerks or other hotel staff. Just because a local point of interest is a short distance away doesn't mean it's safe to run there. We've both had encounters with the fringe element of society after being steered into downtrodden parts of town by well-intentioned concierges.

In some cities, local running stores provide hotels maps of popular routes, so ask the concierge if they have anything like that. Better yet, ask if he or she is a runner – you can trust the advice a lot better if they are.

Be flexible: Vacations almost always create daily schedules that vary from your regular routine – especially if you are travelling with kids or other friends. You'll probably have to switch up your regular running times in order to fit in a run. Don't worry about the change – just take advantage of whatever opportunities there are to fit in a short workout.

Sightsee on the run: In many cities, you can check out local attractions, visit historic districts, or tour scenic parks wearing nothing more than your running shoes. Sometimes a quick early morning run will help you decide what to visit with family or friends later. You'll know the best route, where the restaurants are, or where the best views are. And let's face it – sometimes, there's not much to those local attractions other than what's visible on the surface anyway. So even if you don't spend an hour gawking at the world's largest ball of mud, you can still come home and tell people that you saw it.

Join a race: Occasionally it's fun to see how you match up against the local competition – so if you were able to find a race in your pre-vacation research, we'd definitely recommend signing up. Racing against strangers is far less predictable than running in your hometown races, where you often know before the race even starts how high you'll place in your age group based on whose cars are in the parking lot. You might enjoy some nice post-race food or make some new acquaintances as well.

The next time you travel out of town, instead of bailing on your training plans, use them to enhance the overall experience instead. It's relatively easy to plan for, and the results can be very rewarding.

SOCIAL COMMENTARY: TACKLING ISSUES ONE MILE AT A TIME

"Insurance companies can base their premium rates on physical fitness tests like the ones that used to be given in grade schools. Cardiovascular fitness is the most important predictor of overall health – and if you struggle with a 2-mile test, chances are that your health is lousy. People can be recertified every 2 or 3 years - just like smog inspections for their cars - where an independent timer verifies their 2-mile time, and insurance rates would correspond to their speed. Would that make you take your fitness more seriously?"

"It only takes a matter of minutes before the discarded shirts are claimed by spectators – the majority of whom are the homeless population. It's a bonanza morning for people who sleep on the streets, as shirts rain down like manna from heaven."

Full Disclosure

The excitement of a marathon isn't merely about who crosses the finish line first. There's a whole set of "races within the race" – competitions between people fighting for awards in various subcategories – that are at the heart of the event.

For example, at the Big Sur Marathon, awards are given to the fastest runner in each five-year age group. They are also given for top masters (over 40) runner, Clydesdales (men over 195 lbs), Athenas (women over 150 lbs), active duty military runners, Monterey County residents, as well as denizens of cold weather climates (because they presumably have a harder time training for an April event.)

Strangely, most runners never really know who they're competing against – which leads to some odd conversations during the final miles. A seemingly innocent question of "So, where are you from?" is actually a disguised query as to whether the person is in the Monterey County category. And while it's seemingly more awkward to ask someone's age or (God forbid) weight in the middle of a race, we wouldn't put it past some hyper-competitive runners.

That's why we're proposing that running events adopt a policy that triathlons have used for years: writing each competitor's age on his or her calf. That way, each runner would know the age of everybody in the field around them, and know when they were passing (or getting passed by) someone in the same category.

It's a simple detail that could have an enormous impact on the competitive dynamic of a race. Sometimes there's no better motivation to get through the tough final miles than to know you're locked in a close race for a category award; a primal instinct kicks in when you know you're getting passed by someone of the same age, or even worse, someone that is older. On some level, everyone likes to know where they stand among their chronological peers.

The same thing could be done for the other categories: for instance, "MC" for Monterey County, or a big horseshoe for Clydesdales and Athenas. Sure, the writing on the calf could get pretty crowded, but this information is too valuable to neglect.

Furthermore, everybody knows that when it comes to race performance, age is usually only part of the story. So why stop there? Why can't we write other pertinent information on our legs, so everyone understands exactly who they're going up against?

Here some examples of what we'd like to see on the calves of other runners in our next race, and what the markings might indicate about each person's ability:

37: Age. We need this for obvious reasons.

M or S: Married or single. Does being married make someone a better runner? On one hand, marriage usually implies a time commitment (at least that's what we're told). On the other, it helps to have a support person during strenuous training periods. So this detail is a bit of a wash. But what if we could have…

HM or TM: For "Happy Marriage" or "Troubled Marriage." Wouldn't a happy runner train more effectively than a stressed-out one? Or does the person in a bad marriage spend extra time out on the roads to avoid conflict?

(You know what? Let's just leave marriage out of it – there are way too many variables. But there's no question about…)

3: Number of kids. Put it this way – which woman are you more impressed by: a 38-minute 10K runner with "0" on her calf, or a 41-minute runner with a "4" there? And we haven't even mentioned the women with an "S" (single) as well as a "2" (kids) – they deserve some sort of prize just for showing up with matching socks on.

FT or PT: Full-time or part-time job. This is the eternal working man's (or woman's) complaint: that if he didn't have to work so many hours per week, he'd have more time for training, and would perform better in races. We could further break this down into ML (manual labor) or CDJ (cushy desk job), but that might resemble classism, and we're afraid that somebody might get sued.

Anyway, we'd bet that most of those FT guys probably wouldn't feel nearly as bad about being passed by someone with either PT or U (unemployed) on his calf.

SLWP: Still Lives with Parents. Honestly, we don't know how this affects performance, but at least it would give us a chuckle while we're getting passed by that mama's boy or girl, particularly if they had a high age number.

Clearly, there are all sorts of benefits to knowing this information in running events. In fact – it's such a refreshing idea, why don't we consider a similar system with our everyday lives?

Take your workplace, for instance. Wouldn't it be great if your co-workers wore labels with this type of personal information? (This is where the idea stumbles a bit, because except for strippers and lifeguards, most people's calves aren't visible at work. But we could come up with some alternative – name tags, patches, lapel pins, something. There's got to be a way.)

You would know how many years away your boss is from retirement age, and exactly how young his hood ornament receptionist is. HM-3 guys wouldn't feel as much pressure to match productivity with the S guy who starts putting in 60-hour work weeks. And that SLWP thing would be just as funny.

Now imagine if all businesses did this. When you go out for coffee, you would know the relationship status of that cute barista you make up reasons to buy lattes from four days per week. You'd know the real age of your hairdresser who perennially claims she's 39. And you might be more tolerant if you're on the receiving end of rude customer service from the TM woman at the bagel shop.

The possibilities are endless, and generally beneficial. Over a period of time, we'd all come to experience heightened awareness and mutual understanding of those around us.

And all it would take is a little bit of temporary body marking.

Fighting Obesity

The Centers for Disease Control recently sponsored the first "Weight of the Nation" conference, where it was announced that the medical cost of obesity in the United States each year is $147 BILLION. Almost one-third of American adults are officially categorized as obese, with rates in many (mostly Southern) states approaching 40%. Even Oprah Winfrey is overweight again.

What's the solution? The CDC has a standard laundry list of recommendations to stop the obesity epidemic, but it's the same things we've been told for years: healthier food choices, lower caloric intake, more physical exercise. This is all old news, yet obesity rates continue to rise.

So we'd like to suggest some changes in perspective for all of us – the first of which is to encourage support from selected "influencers" who can connect with large numbers of people.

One such program is right in our backyard: the Big Sur International Marathon's Just Run program. As we've said before, the formula for what works is no secret: less food, more activity. Just Run instills this lesson in elementary school children, and gives them opportunities to make healthy choices from a very early age. Good habits start young.

Our educational system can go one step further and make physical education mandatory in all schools. Programs can be supported with minimal cost, even at schools without a dedicated PE teacher; all it takes is a committed volunteer to get students walking or jogging every day.

Healthy activity is just as important to our kids' quality of life as art and music and great literature.

Parents play a key role as well. We should teach our kids to be participants in athletics instead of spectators. Modern-day sporting events (and their accompanying advertisers) promote tailgating, beer drinking, and pigging out on unhealthy food just as much as they inspire sandlot games and schoolyard shoot-arounds. It's our job as parents to remind kids that the fun of sports is in doing, not watching.

Professional sports leagues can even get in on the act. Imagine if championship sporting events had associated running races, like a marathon on Super Bowl Sunday, or a 5K before the local pro golf tournament. Have the pro athletes make an appearance beforehand, or provide discount tickets to the big event to encourage participation in the fitness activity.

Another approach is to borrow a page from the anti-smoking playbook, and make it cost-prohibitive for people to be unhealthy.

For instance, what if you had to pay for exorbitant cable or Internet screen time in the same way that you pay for excess usage of water or electricity? Since obsessive screen watching makes people less active and obese – how about creating a graduated "sin tax" beyond a certain threshold?

Insurance companies can base their premium rates on physical fitness tests like the ones that used to be given in grade schools. Cardiovascular fitness is the most important predictor of overall health – and if you struggle with a 2-mile test, chances are that your health is lousy. People can be recertified every 2 or 3 years - just like smog inspections for their cars - where an independent timer verifies their 2-mile time, and insurance rates would correspond to their speed. Would that make you take your fitness more seriously?

These ideas may sound crazy – but that's indicative of a larger problem, which is complacency to let things carry on the same way they're currently going. If prioritizing our health continues to be seen as the "counterculture" approach, we're in for far more troubling costs in the days ahead – both from a health standpoint, and a financial one.

Olympic Lessons

Sometimes, a race is just a race. Other times, it can reveal something of a person's character – and not just for the athletes, but for those watching them as well. Last month's Olympic track meet provided one such instance of the latter category.

I (Donald) figured that watching the meet would be a fantastic opportunity to expose my two older kids to the events, and gauge their respective interest level. My son had just been to a track meet where he raced (well, sort of) in two sprints, and he liked watching the runners race the same distance – 100 meters - that he ran a couple of weeks earlier. My daughter hasn't ever really paid attention to any sports, but she sat on my lap to watch a few races, and understood that her Daddy does the same thing (well, sort of) as the runners on TV.

Despite their generally comparable upbringing, my son and daughter are very dissimilar creatures, and view the world quite differently in many ways. Watching the Athens Games together made some of these disparities even more evident.

My 6-year-old son is a pure logician, curious to know how things work, constantly analyzing the structure and mechanics of any item or event. He thinks like a scientist, and occasionally misses the forest for the biochemical composition and root structure of each individual tree.

Watching the 100m race from the elevated camera angle, he spotted the trackside camera moving along the railing beside the runners, and recognized the shots that came from this particular camera as they were interspersed in the broadcast. He wanted to know how they started the camera rolling down the track, and if they adjusted the speed of it to account for faster or slower runners. He also asked if the aerial shots of the stadium came from a blimp or a helicopter. He wondered how the runners know where to place the starting blocks before the start. (I felt bad for not knowing the answers – because these seemed like awfully good questions. As a Dad, I really should learn these things.)

Later, he asked if anyone had tried banking the curves of the track to make it easier for runners to turn when they are going fast (actually, I knew this one! The answer is yes…indoor tracks are built this way). Basically, he was turning the Olympic track meet into an episode of *Modern Marvels.*

Having just recently discovered the concept of competition, his typical pattern during races was first to ask, "Is that guy winning?" and if the answer was yes, then say, "That's the one I'm cheering for." Always a winner, this kid.

By contrast, my 3-year-old daughter is naturally considerate, compassionate, and nurturing - at such a level that it frequently eclipses that of her own parents. She has the same powers of observation as her brother, only for different things.

As she sat in my lap watching various races, she noticed the many different colors of the runners' skin, which led to a nice discussion about diversity of cultures and ethnicities. (Incidentally, she seemed more attuned to this than NBC, who somehow didn't notice that Jeremy Wariner was the first white American to win a sprint medal since 1964. Are we so politically sensitive that we aren't allowed to mention this? It seems like a great talking point for breaking down racial stereotypes. Sorry, I'm ranting.).

When the runners were introduced before each race, my daughter wanted to learn their names. In a couple of women's races, she asked if a particularly muscular female was a boy or a girl (and stunningly, she was acutely insightful; one of the women she questioned was later stripped of a medal for steroid use). She asked if any the women who were running were also mommies. She probably didn't even realize that the runners were racing, but after they finished she often commented, "They look tired."

Of course, I'm just as susceptible to natural bias as my children are. As the women's 400m hurdles race unfolded, the TV commentators marveled at the inspirational performance of the Greek champion who was carried to victory by a delirious home crowd, and stood atop the podium for one of the most emotional medal ceremonies of the Games. Watching the same race at home, I was thinking to myself, "Hmm … here is a woman who currently runs the 400m hurdles faster than she ran the open (no hurdles) 400m one year ago, who has become dramatically faster in her event in an extremely short period of time, and is a teammate of two other Greek runners who had just been banned from the competition for steroid use. Are we just supposed to believe that these facts are entirely coincidental?"

My cynical mind just couldn't submit to the apparent splendor of the scene – but to my credit, I kept such thoughts to myself while my daughter admired the Greek runner's long blond hair, "Like I have. And like Cinderella has." I didn't have the heart to tell her that this particular Cinderella probably had a higher testosterone level than most princes she knows.

It's always interesting to discover how different people can view the same event at the same time, and make completely different observations and conclusions about it based on the inherent filters through which we see the world. While it might seem a bit unusual that such discrepancies would bubble to the surface during a track meet, in my house a running event could be the backdrop for just about anything.

Besides, the Olympics are clearly a special occasion. I mean … how many other shows can a compulsively analytical boy, a romantic touchy-feely girl, and their overly jaded father all watch together with equal enjoyment? I guess that's one of the things that makes the Olympic track meet special: it has something for everybody.

You Go Girls!

Beginning in 2004, the Los Angeles Marathon staged an annual "Battle of the Sexes," giving the elite female runners a 15-minute head start over the elite males. The first person, male or female, to reach the finish line received an extra $100,000 in bonus money in addition to the normal first-place payday.

The Battle doesn't determine which is the better-performing gender on race day, and it doesn't speak to whether women are better runners than men. The idea was to have the media focus separately on the female runners, to increase the profile of women's distance running. However, it was also something of a publicity stunt, which some detractors say compromised the real value and beauty of the race.

(Truth be told, we'd like to see a different method of generating artificial excitement in a marathon. How about having the men and women start at opposite ends of the course, and run the race in different directions? Imagine how cool it would be as the lead packs of men and women approached each other - it would look like the final battle scene from Braveheart. We could call it Extreme Marathoning, or Demolition Derby Marathon. It would certainly make for good television.)

To purists, there's not much sense in resorting to gimmicks like pitting men against women in a marathon. Indeed, one of the best things about running – either in training or racing - is the opportunity to spend quality time with members of the opposite sex, developing a mutual respect for each other without the stress of competing amongst ourselves.

At almost any race, the ensemble of men and women struggling together is a model of gender equality. There are very few places in life where men and women compete on truly equal footing - but in running, they each face the same distance, the same weather conditions, and race against the same clock. It's a situation that many women enjoy – and one of the best developments over the past several years has been the significant increase in female marathoners stepping up to the task. Today, most American marathons see a nearly equal percentage of male and female participants on the starting line.

All things considered, female marathoners actually accomplish a lot more than the men who race alongside them. Let's be honest: it's typically much more difficult for women to train on a daily basis than their male counterparts.

Both of us have always had the luxury of supportive wives to watch our kids while we spend hours on the roads and trails. Many of our female training partners don't have the same luxury, and typically have to juggle their workouts along with family responsibilities and career obligations. Some have spouses who also work, while others are single parents dependent on child care just to get outside to train.

Females also have a monopoly on the childbirth process, which we hear is less than pleasant. Dramatic body transformations such as weight fluctuation, muscle soreness, cardiovascular compromise, and rampant hormonal changes throughout pregnancy and for more than a year after childbirth can certainly limit one's ability to log consistent mileage in training. It's no mystery why most elite female athletes postpone having children until their competitive racing days are over.

We recognize the extra hurdles many women overcome just to participate in our sport, and we have enormous respect for their accomplishments, regardless of their speed. We love seeing our female friends at local races, and we hope to see many more of them in the future. It doesn't interest us to compare our fastest times to theirs, or to worry about who crosses the finish line first – because that's really not the point of our sport.

We'd rather run alongside them, and then celebrate our achievements together when the race is over.

Fitness Made Simple

Running is a true grassroots sport, without need for world-famous professionals or high-profile celebrities to stimulate widespread interest. Unfortunately, the same can't be said for many home-workout programs.

For example, I (Donald) can't get away from John Basedow. Almost every time my television is on, I see a commercial for one of his home workout videos. He promises that by following the exercise routines and nutritional tips - that he himself practices! - you can sculpt a physique similar to his in just a short period of time.

The commercials have testimonials from people who have turned their lives around, saying things like "you can't put a price on this kind of happiness," just before they show the $30-40 price per video that Basedow puts on this kind of happiness.

Yet there's something about Basedow's physique that looks a bit freakish to me. He has a big head of frosted, feathered hair atop an obnoxiously muscular torso that is polished as smooth as marble. His muscle definition seems almost too pronounced, like a grown-up action figure, with a suspicious "cosmetic pectoral implants" appearance. The dime-store special effects, such as cartoon flames rising on either side of him during the *Fat Burning Workout* commercial, only add to the surrealism.

I often can't decide whether to be disgusted or amused by the constant barrage of Basedow commercials. The titles of his videos, such as *6-pack Abs, AM/PM workout,* and *Fat Burning Workout,* are clichéd and completely generic. His corny descriptions of "no tricky dance moves, no high-impact gyrations" often make me wince.

What always strikes me is that he's identified as "fitness celebrity John Basedow." Now, the only time *I've* ever heard of this guy is when I'm watching his ads. For what, exactly, is he recognized as a celebrity - for saturating the cable market with cheesy infomercials? Does he hold some record for the number of appearances on television without a shirt?

All in all, he just doesn't impress me. Even among other workout-video gurus, he doesn't seem that remarkable. Personally, I'd put my money on Tae-Bo instructor Billy Blanks to lay the smack down on Basedow any day.

Initially I thought Basedow was just a one-man cottage industry in California, until I watched Tony Kornheiser make fun of him on ESPN's talk show *Pardon the Interruption.* Knowing that *PTI* tapes in Washington, D.C., I realized that Basedow was saturating both coasts with his spiel.

So with California and the Northeast covered, I had to know- what about the red states? I called my Mom in Colorado. Sure enough, she immediately knew who I was asking about, calling him "that 30-minute ab guy." She even threw in that, "it seems like he's on TV all the time" without my prompting.

The thought occurred to me – could it be that *this* is the uniter our country has been looking for over the past five years? It seems unfathomable, but perhaps it speaks to the underpinnings of our country. After all, despite so many moral and political differences, Americans can at least find common ground in our shared desire for washboard abs, right?

Begrudgingly, I figured I had to give Basedow some credit. He has managed to get his product and message across to millions of Americans, at all hours of the day and night. I'm not sure how wealthy he has become, but at a minimum, he must make enough money to pay for the thousands of nationwide commercial spots he buys.

I guess from a runner's standpoint, the thing that annoys me the most is that one of us didn't think of this idea first. I mean ... "fitness made simple"? Isn't that the definition of running? How much more simple does it get than repeatedly placing one foot in front of the other?

Running doesn't have tricky dance moves or high-impact gyrations, either. It's the best fat-burning exercise around. It can be done in the AM or the PM. It can help you shed all of that stuff covering up the six-pack abdominal muscles. To borrow a phrase from Basedow's ads, running has been "bringing real results to real people" for decades. Somehow I feel like we runners missed the boat on this potential marketing scheme.

Think of the possibilities. I could sell a 30-minute video of me doing a workout routine that I actually do myself: running. I could film myself on some scenic beach, like Denise Austin does for her workout videos. Even on a limited expense budget, I could simply record myself running on a treadmill, saying a lot of self-affirming psychobabble.

After I get off the treadmill, I'll make myself a smoothie, the nutritional component of my workout program. Do this once a day for 3 months - and oh, by the way, don't eat any junk food either. Soon, the pounds will start melting away, even while you sleep!

My training partners can testify about how much they've improved over the years, and how their self-esteem is worth far more than the price of the videos. I'll call myself a "running celebrity" and charge $30 per video for this stuff - or better yet, I could hire someone attractive to run on the treadmill (and pose in flattering positions in the ads), and charge $40 each. Start airing ads on cable TV, and there's all kinds of potential here.

Or...maybe not. I guess one of the things I like best about running is that it's not gimmicky, and doesn't rely on some guru selling us a newly developed secret technique or method. It's not a fitness fad that needs celebrity endorsements to prolong its fifteen minutes in the popular consciousness. It is unquestionably effective in producing beneficial results.

I like the body that running gives me, even if I can't bounce a quarter off my stomach or crack a walnut between my buttocks. Best of all, I like the way it makes me feel. Being a runner gives me simultaneous mental and physical fitness; fitness made very, very simple.

Chemical Games

Over the past several years, Marion Jones, Justin Gatlin, and Floyd Landis have been among the most celebrated names in sports. Today, they are merely the latest performance enhancement drug suspects in a long tradition of infamy.

We are embarrassed that our sport, which is so fundamentally simple, has been tarnished by drug scandals like so many others. However, we're also proud that running and cycling have the most rigorous drug testing policies around. But sometimes, imperfect tests merely add to the confusion.

This won't be your typical article about drugs. It's not that we don't care. We take the issue very seriously. It's an admission that we have absolutely no idea what the best solution might be.

One school of thought says that we should legalize everything for competition. If you want to use HGH or EPO or synthetic testosterone, or do some blood doping, go right ahead. If you want to roll the dice and risk your long-term health, that's your business.

It doesn't appear to be much of a moral dilemma for many athletes to use drugs to gain a competitive advantage. We suspect that one reason they cheat is because they believe most of their competitors are doing the same. The financial rewards for victory can be tremendous motivators, no matter how you reach the top. You can see how this could potentially spiral into a situation where everybody's juicing, because nobody would want to be stuck with the equivalent of bringing only a knife to a gun fight.

So it's not too difficult to envision a future competition where all the athletes are on some drug or another. One sport – bodybuilding – has gone down this road, to the point where they hold two separate competitions: there's a Mr. Universe for drug users, and a "Mr. Natural Universe" for anyone else.

In fact, many people will tell you this "everybody's juiced" situation is exactly what we have in track and cycling today. The only difference with bodybuilding is that they don't ask us to pretend otherwise.

What if running formally adopted such a policy? Instead of merely having the best athletic ability, competitors would also strive to have the most potent pharmacological cocktail on board before their peak races.

They would be dependent on chemists and lab geeks to achieve their success. Imagine every sprinter's posse with one skinny, bespectacled guy in a short-sleeve plaid shirt with a pocket protector roaming around trying to look cool with the rest of the group. If nothing else, it would provide some comedic irony.

Think about it – who got teased and beat up more in high school than the kids in chemistry club? And weren't the jocks usually the ones doing most of the bullying? And now those two groups would be pairing off in the strangest oddball symbiotic relationships this side of Michael Jackson and Lisa Marie Presley.

The chemists would actually have the upper hand in these partnerships. They would be too valuable to the athlete to be fired – because the chemist could then go and tell everybody else what particular designer drugs the athlete was on. And the athlete knows he or she won't succeed without the help of a good lab geek.

The chemistry dudes could totally revel in this, and do all kinds of trash talking with the sprinters. Between events at track meets, they can congregate on the infield to gossip about their athletes, draw formulas in the dirt and swap periodic table jokes. They might even encounter chemistry groupies wanting to make "covalent bonds" with them after the meets.

Over time, the chemists would get the same rock star treatment the athletes get. The better ones would sign exclusive rights contracts with companies like Nike or Adidas and become millionaires. Scores of little kids will dream of a career in laboratory science, and of growing up to compete at the "Chemical Games," where the torch is an enormous Bunsen burner. The best chemistry students coming out of grad school could be drafted by professional teams and awarded lucrative signing bonuses.

If you're a career chemist, where's the downside to any of this?

Realistically, we know this isn't going to happen, and we suppose that's for the good. Sports have an inherently noble premise: that athletes are testing the limits of their God-given talents through nothing more than hard work and determination. And despite our jaded outlook, it's a premise we're completely in favor of defending.

Yes, the tests are light years behind the cheaters, but that doesn't mean we should stop the effort. It's just going to take a very long time before the priority (and money) given to testing is equal to the money that changes hands among the top athletes and corporations in every sport.

Until then, most sports will continue to have an anemic system of testing (One time per year for a baseball player? Spare us.), and they'll continue to profess that they're doing everything in their power to rid sports of doping.

All of the top-level athletes will emphatically assert that they are completely clean, and fans will believe what they want to believe about each athlete based on his or her carefully crafted image.

Meanwhile, none of us will ever know for sure if the next heroes like Marion Jones or Floyd Landis are true champions, or merely another example of all that's wrong with sports. And that is the true tragedy.

How Young is Too Young?

As you're reading this, 13-year-old Jordan Romero of Big Bear, CA, is bivouacked at 22,000' on the slopes of Mount Everest, preparing for a summit bid that would make him the youngest person ever to stand on the world's highest peak.

Despite his age, Romero is no novice; he's climbed to the highest points on five other continents, and has more mountaineering experience than many "tourist climbers" who pay for guided expeditions on Everest. However, his attempt has been met with equal parts praise and outrage by experienced mountain climbers. Some see him as a role model for a generation of unhealthy, overweight kids. Others consider him a poster boy for reckless ambition and misguided parental prioritization.

The question is simple, but the answer is incredibly complex: how old should kids be before taking on extreme athletic challenges?

The running community grapples with a similar dilemma – albeit on a less dramatic scale than mountain climbing – in considering at what age children should be permitted to enter marathons or ultramarathons. Nearly every race today has a minimum age requirement, but in the 1970s, very young runners were somewhat commonplace at major marathons.

Prior to instituting a minimum age of 18 in 1981, the New York City Marathon saw approximately 75 runners aged 8 to 13 cross its finish line in the late 1970s. The Los Angeles Marathon's Students Run LA program annually trains kids ages 12 to 18 to finish the event. Locally, the Big Sur Marathon's minimum age is 16 – although in an interesting twist, its medical director ran his first marathon at age 13, and his first ultra at age 14. Last month, four 16-year-olds successfully completed Big Sur's challenging 26.2-mile Highway 1 course.

So how young is too young? Is 12 or 16 more risky than 18? What about 10? Or 8? And what exactly is the rationale for any of these guidelines?

The American Academy of Pediatricians recommends that runners focus on shorter events like the 10K or half-marathon until age 18. A group called the International Marathon Medical Directors Association cites the AAP guideline in its own recommendation for an 18-year-old age requirement. Curiously, the standards are based as much on psychological considerations as they are on physiology.

For example, it's true that kids with developing bones and muscles are highly susceptible to overuse injuries with endurance running – but this is a consequence for many adults who train excessively as well. Children's bodies aren't as adept at thermoregulation, leaving them susceptible to heat-related problems during a race – but the bodies of novice marathoners are equally unprepared in this regard. Overall, the physical risks of the marathon for youngsters aren't significantly greater than those for adults.

Instead, the primary concern expressed by most running authorities, as well as grown-ups who started as extremely young distance runners, is that kids might be trying the marathon for the wrong reasons, and might burn out on running relatively early in life. From a standpoint of promoting lifelong health, it's always better for runners of any age to build up to the marathon gradually, over a period of years instead of weeks. And if parental pressures are any factor in a child entering the marathon, the likelihood of he or she continuing as an independent adult is fairly low.

In the end, every situation is unique to the individuals involved, in running just as it is in mountain climbing. There will always be precocious kids who are physically gifted and genuinely self-driven enough to take on such challenges, and there will always be some who are better off building up to such things patiently. The only things we can wish for Jordan Romero or any other young athletes are for them always to be safe, have fun, and develop a passion for healthy activity that lasts a lifetime.

**Postscript: Jordan Romero reached the summit of Mount Everest on May 22, 2010.*

Infomercial Fitness

From time to time, both of us have battled recurring injuries. The standard advice injured runners always hear is to take some rest.

Unfortunately, we both happen to be terribly impatient. We get antsy when we can't go running. So during our "rest" periods, we look to other forms of exercise to stay in shape until we can hit the roads again.

Fortunately we have television access for our indoor cross-training. Whenever we're pedaling away at a stationary bike or tugging on a rowing machine, we channel surf through the countless infomercials promising a fast lane to fitness. (Unless of course we come across a *Girls Gone Wild* infomercial, in which case we immediately stop surfing – but not pedaling.)

We're amazed at how much we didn't know about fitness before we started watching early morning television. Sure, running is the easiest and fastest way to get in shape, but apparently it isn't the sexiest.

Now we have some better alternatives. Here then is our money-back guaranteed recommendation for anyone looking to achieve peak physical fitness:

You have a DVD player, right? Buy several DVDs that you can alternate from day to day in the comfort and privacy of your own home. Monday can be *Yoga Booty Ballet*, hosted by fitness superstars Teigh and Gillian. Hollywood celebrities use it to flex, firm, and burn. This workout seems primarily aimed at women, but men would certainly enjoy watching Teigh and Gillian work their booties. Like we said, you're in the privacy of home.

On Tuesday try Chalene's *Turbo Jam Workout*. You can lose 10 pounds and 10 inches in 10 days while learning calorie-busting kickboxing and dance moves. And Chalene's not bad to look at, either.

Wednesday would be the classic, the pioneer: John Basedow's *Fitness Made Simple*. John cares about you. Just do John's workouts and follow John's nutrition recommendations and any man will undoubtedly end up looking like John. Single women will land themselves a man that looks like John, so everybody wins.

On Thursday do the *Inside and Out 6 Week Body Makeover* with Michael Thurmond. You can sleep in a little, too, because you'll only need 18 minutes for the body sculpting routine. You'll be able to eat more, exercise less, and get fit – guaranteed. Michael is a master body sculptor who has transformed the bodies of countless celebrities.

Then again, you can work out with real celebrities on the remaining three days of the week.

Supermodel Elle McPherson and less-than-super actor Patrick Duffy are spokespeople for *Supreme Pilates.* Note that it is "supreme," meaning it must be WAY better than that plain old *Winsor Pilates* crap that Daisy Fuentes sells. But don't play favorites – give each of them one day of the week. Besides, how exciting would it be to have both Elle and Daisy in your living room? It's the kind of thing guys dream about.

Don't think that Sunday is a rest day, because we've reserved that day for our favorite workout, Billy Blanks' *Tae-Bo Boot Camp.* You'll transform your body and mind, and blast into shape in just 7 days. Have you seen Billy? Would you argue with him? Us either.

So you've got your indoor workouts covered. What if you want some fresh air? In that case, we recommend that you park the cars outside and start filling your garage with exercise equipment. No, it's not really outside, but this way you're protected from the harsh wind and rain. And sunlight.

Sure, it can get quite expensive, but if you are serious about total fitness, you absolutely need this equipment. Start with the Bowflex Extreme, for as little as $20/month. You'll still be paying for it six years from now, but by then you'll have the body you always wanted. You're worth it!

If that's not your style, how about the Total Gym? In just 6 to 8 minutes a day, you can look like Chuck Norris or Christie Brinkley. All this time, did you think Christie was just naturally beautiful? If it weren't for the Total Gym, she'd be just as frumpy as the rest of us.

Leave room in the garage for abdominal machines. Those old fashioned sit-ups and crunches are for chumps. Work your abs into a frenzy with the Ab-doer, Ab-blaster, Ab-Lounger, RED (Rotational Exercise Device), or (our favorite) the Torso Tiger. Or if eight minutes per day is too much commitment, just buy the Slendertone Flex Ab-Belt, which you simply wear and go about your daily routine, with no exercise needed.

Got all that? Your exercise regimen is now complete. Oh, wait – there's one more thing. Read the fine print on all of these revolutionary programs:

Results may vary. Advertised results not typical. You may be less successful. And of course, *Best results are achieved by using this product along with a consistent program of sensible diet and traditional exercise.*

You know, traditional exercise … like running.

Come to think of it, being injured sucks. We'd much rather save our money, and just get back out on the trails and roads.

Judges? We Don't Need No Stinking Judges!

I (Donald) generally love the Olympics. There's really no more inspirational and uplifting sporting event in the world.

And while I prefer the Summer Games with their track and field events, I've really been enjoying these Winter Games in … um, what exactly is the name of that city? I always thought it was Turin, as in "Shroud of Turin." But NBC is determined to call it *Torino*, like the Ford car that Starsky and Hutch drove.

(Did I miss a protocol change somewhere? Should we Americans now refer to the Italian capital as *Roma*, or the city with canals as *Venezia*? Or is NBC just trying to sound more sophisticated? If somebody could clarify this, I'd appreciate it. Maybe I just need to watch more Geography Bees.)

Anyway, I've been watching these Olympics, enthralled by the speed of lugers and downhill skiers, and awed by the power of the speed skaters.

I became a fan of cross-country skiing during the 2002 Games, after watching the 4 × 10K relay competition between Italy and Norway decided by less than a second, and learning that these same two countries have finished within a second of each other in each of the previous two Olympic Games. They've got a rivalry going that makes the Red Sox and Yankees look like Little Leaguers by comparison.

Invariably however, several winter sports don't hold my interest for very long – snowboarding, aerial jumping, and moguls to name a few.

The marquis sport of the Games, figure skating, impresses me with its grace and athleticism, but it's hard to see it as an honest competition in light of recent judging scandals. Put it this way: any time the Russian mob is involved with determining the winner, the results have to be viewed somewhat skeptically.

So here's my litmus test for following a sport in these Winter Games: any event where the result depends on style points, or scores given by judges, is far less attractive to me than those involving traditional competition.

Clearly, my obsession for running has biased my perception and appreciation of other sports. Events where athletes or teams compete head-to-head, or race against the clock, just seem inherently purer and more exciting.

One of the greatest aspects of running is its fundamental nature: go from here to there as fast as you can, using only your body. The clock tells us precisely how well we perform, and exactly how we fare in comparison to everyone else. There is nothing abstract or biased about our finishing place. Watch any local 5K or 10K race, and you will witness the most genuine form of competition anywhere to be found.

At the Winter Games, that notion gets turned on its head – and even some sports that appear objective at first glance have a subjective component that feels unnatural. For example, doesn't it seem obvious that for ski jumping, the winner would be the one who flies the farthest? However, the jumpers are also given style points based on their landings - which, unless someone completely crashes, all look remarkably similar to me. So instead of comparing the distances, the jumpers are given a composite "score" and ranked accordingly. Huh?

Thank goodness this standard doesn't apply to running. Some of the greatest runners in history looked like miserable wretches at the time of their highest achievement.

The great Czech runner Emil Zatopek, who won three gold medals at the 1952 Helsinki Olympics, often ran with his head cocked to one side, with his tongue hanging out of his mouth, and his eyes bulging from their sockets. A famous description of him was that he looked like a man with a noose around his neck.

American Steve Prefontaine ran with his head wrenched backward, flung his arms in every direction, and had an expression of sheer agony during every one of his races. He tried to decide races based on who had the most guts, frequently defeating opponents who ran much more gracefully.

There is a long list of elite runners who during the course of a race have thrown up, relieved themselves, or become bruised and bloody in pursuit of their goal. Consider how revolting it would be (even more so than the actual throwing up, relieving themselves, etc) if their accomplishments were considered secondary to those runners who looked more sophisticated while running more slowly.

This aspect of running applies to us amateurs also. As a physical therapist, I spend a lot of time watching people walk, analyzing the biomechanics of their stride. During training runs or long races, when my mind drifts, I instinctively assess the form of runners around me.

I can attest that there are a lot of ugly runners out there. Feet slapping the ground, elbows flailing, heads lolling all about - it's easy to find these and many more gait abnormalities if you look around the crowd at your next 10K. However, many of these weirdoes run extraordinarily fast race times.

There are also a lot of ugly *sounding* runners, whose groaning and gasping keep the medical personnel at aid stations on high alert during races. But those of us running near them typically don't even give a second thought to their clamorous efforts. The great thing is, it doesn't really matter what we look like or sound like as we race.

Our pleasure and satisfaction come not from our presentation, but in attaining the tangible results for which we strive. Best of all, it doesn't take a panel of judges to tell us if we have succeeded.

The Value of Fitness

There's an old saying to "put your money where your mouth is;" more recently, sports agent Jerry Maguire famously screamed "SHOW ME THE MONEY!!" Both phrases reflect the same point: the way people and businesses spend money is indicative of what's truly important to them. To a lesser extent, it also reflects who their role models are.

For example, consider how the American public and corporate America value fitness and athletic achievement. "Fitness" gets a lot of lip service - but when it comes time to show the money, some stark truths emerge, especially when you study the differences between running and golf, two common recreational activities with similar demographics but vastly different financial rewards. I (Mike) have had first-hand experience in both of these groups, and the contrasts are amazing.

Before I turned to running as a healthy and competitive outlet when I was nearly 40, I was a pretty fair golfer. I played intercollegiate golf at U.C. Berkeley, and participated in regional U.S. Open qualifying twice. I was on a "what's up" basis with Tom Watson and Johnny Miller. My handicap was scratch. I held some course records and won a few amateur tournaments.

So why didn't I turn pro? Because I was smart enough to know I didn't have "It." Golf requires the utmost patience and control over your emotions as well as tremendous technical skill. Some people have It, and others don't. Virtually every top golf pro started playing as a pre-teen, in a controlled environment, with a watchful father figure who was either a professional golfer or very knowledgeable about the sport – but there's something intangible that sets the great ones apart. The anointed ones like Tiger Woods had It very early. I didn't and I knew it. Desire, hard work, and effort couldn't overcome lack of It.

My primary athletic calling over the past 20 years has been running, but I often think about my decision to abandon competitive golf. In particular, watching golf's U.S. Open every June causes me to become maudlin and a bit upset.

What brings on the bitterness? Start by comparing the numbers of participants in the two sports. According to the National Golf Foundation, there are 28 million golfers in the United States who played one round or more last year. Slightly less than 2 million played 100 times or more. About 600,000 of these frequent golfers are over 50. Golfers spent $3.2 billion on golf merchandise or related purchases.

Contrast this with running: according to Running USA there are 34.9 million runners in the United States who run regularly, and slightly over 10 million who run 100 times a year. About 2 million of these frequent runners are over 50. Runners spent $5.1 billion on running-related purchases. Thus, there are more runners in America than golfers, and they spend more money on their chosen activity.

Now compare the prize money in the two sports. In 1998, Hale Irwin was the top senior golfer in the country, winning $2.8 million in tournament money and well more than that in endorsements. The 100th place senior was Jack Lewis with about $35,000 in tournament winnings. 2004's leading senior money winner was Craig Stadler - affectionately nicknamed The Walrus - with an estimated $5.5 million in total earnings.

In 1997 and 1998, shortly after turning 50, I traveled throughout the United States to race against the best senior competition in the country, and was ranked in the top 5 every year from 1997 to 2001. Very few races offer prize money, and the highest-paying race in the country paid $200 for the senior winner – an amount that Craig Stadler might spend on lunch. My total combined race winnings in those 5 years, even with several wins, were $1,350. Needless to say, no one was beating down my door with endorsement opportunities either.

None of my competitors had a nickname like "The Walrus." They were all gazelles. Several former Olympians and major marathon winners, such as Frank Shorter and Bill Rodgers, compete as seniors. The others are hard-working anonymous no-names like Sal Vasquez, Jim Gorman, Don Porteus, Jan Frisby, and Nolan Shaheed. On the women's side, Shirley Matson, Joan Ottoway, Kathy Martin, and Sister Marion Irvine are incredible athletes over age 50. Have you ever heard of them?

Athletic pundits sometimes ask if golfers are truly athletes. I know from experience that playing golf at the highest levels is extremely exhausting. I've run 27 marathons, but I have never been as physically and emotionally drained as when I participated in a competitive medal play event at Spyglass Hill and Pebble Beach golf course.

Staring at 4 and 5 foot putts all day long can be brutal. The pressure can be overwhelming and it's constant for over 5 hours. Golfers may not be athletes in the sense that runners consider, but their accomplishments are truly remarkable, and the most successful ones are richly rewarded.

The Walrus is swimming in corporate sponsorship and tournament winnings; if you read his press and look at his belly, he eats a lot, drinks his weight in beer, is a wine expert, smokes cigars, and has some anger management issues. He is definitely entertaining to watch, and he plays golf better than any other 50-year-old on the senior tour.

But here's the question…should we as sports fans value his skill and talent more than Jim Gorman's, Nolan Shaheed's or Shirley Matson's? They train every day. They endure physical pain in races that would make the Walrus bellow and flop on the ground. They eat right. They are true role models in terms of healthy lifestyle, motivation, and hard work. They show everyone that we have incredible human potential and that the athletic life has no age limits.

Of course, the great senior runners are not in the competitions for the money, but for fun and the challenge of personal accomplishment. But really, shouldn't their success be valued more than $200 per race? It's a sad observation of where our society puts its money.

Race Shirt Blues

If you're a runner who enters a lot of races, sooner or later you'll get a case of the race shirt blues.

It's standard practice for every race to provide entrants with shirts for doing nothing more than paying the entry fee. Once you accumulate enough shirts to overflow your dresser drawers, some kind of selection hierarchy is implemented, where the oldest or least attractive shirts are cleared out and given to relatives or Goodwill. Only the best and most memorable shirts are saved.

While we don't hesitate to unload such unwanted clothing, the shirts from our favorite races often foster an emotional attachment for us. For many runners, they may provide an identity or sense of pride. Wearing a race shirt is often a statement declaring that we enjoy healthy activities and participating in challenging events.

The more difficult the event, the greater "prestige" factor of the shirt – for example, on the Monterey Peninsula, wearing a Big Sur Marathon shirt is something like a badge of courage and accomplishment. That's why we sometimes feel a bit protective about who should rightfully wear shirts from certain races.

In previous articles we've mentioned a few rules of race shirt etiquette, which have all been scientifically proven to bring disaster upon the naïve runner (OK, not really – but you can trust us). The cardinal rule of juju – that you have to participate in an event before you wear the shirt – is why we're somewhat mystified by people who wear event shirts from other sports which merely advertise their attendance as spectators. This peculiarity seems especially prevalent among the golf community.

Someday, if you want to stir up some trouble, try this: the next time you're in an elevator with someone wearing a U.S. Open golf shirt, ask them how they played. When they look at you like you're an idiot and answer, "Oh, I didn't play, I watched the Open at Pebble Beach," you can say, "Wow … that must have been a lot of work. You should be proud of yourself." (On second thought, maybe you should wait until you're out of the elevator to say this, and then take off running. Don't worry – there's no way that lazy duffer will be able to catch you.)

Here's another game you can play sometime: go to a local mall or shopping center and start looking around for race shirts. On an average day you'll probably see several people wearing the shirt of one race or another. Your task is to guess whether the person wearing the shirt is actually the one who ran the race, or a relative of a runner, or just somebody who shops at thrift stores. This game is harder than you think; many fit-looking people may in fact be imposters, and many with "non-athletic" appearances might be the real deal. Of course, since you'll never actually ask them (we hope), there's no way of keeping an accurate score – but it's a fun diversion nevertheless.

In larger cities, the misuse of race shirts has reached epidemic proportions – as we've each discovered while running in San Francisco during and after the city's annual marathon.

The San Francisco Marathon starts at the Ferry Building and heads along the Embarcadero toward the Golden Gate Bridge. Typically, runners wear their least favorite old race shirt at the start line to keep warm in the early morning cold. They then jettison the extra top somewhere along the Embarcadero as their bodies get warmed up.

It only takes a matter of minutes before the discarded shirts are claimed by spectators – the majority of whom on an early, chilly morning are the homeless population. It's a bonanza morning for people who sleep on the streets, as shirts rain down like manna from heaven. The week after the marathon, it's common to see vagabonds pushing shopping carts and wearing layers of Napa Valley Marathon and Bay to Breakers shirts to keep warm.

This chain of events causes potentially confusing sights for untrained tourists walking along the Embarcadero or Fisherman's Wharf afterward. Someone could look around the sidewalks and store fronts and easily conclude that a lot of local runners have somehow fallen on very hard times. A worse scenario would be if an actual runner collapses on the ground during his routine morning workout, and no one stops to help because he seemingly fits right in with the other nearby derelicts who are also sporting threadbare race shirts.

Incidentally, the same wardrobe tossing ritual happens along beautiful Highway 1 during the Big Sur Marathon – but to their credit, the race organization makes sure that any clothing is picked up by volunteers immediately after the race. Each year, about 15 to 20 large trash bags filled with discarded shirts are brought to a warehouse, and shortly thereafter given to local charities.

As we consider this, maybe the misuse of old race shirts isn't such a bad thing after all. Our discarded clothing provides benefit to other people, whether for basic comforts like warmth, or for bargain hunters who might feel some sense of participation by wearing somebody else's marathon shirt.

In an ideal world, some of those folks would then be motivated to start a running or exercise program of their own. Later on, they'll enter races and receive their own shirts – and once they've done a lot of races and have to weed out the old ones, they'll pay it forward by tossing those old shirts on to some new owners. While such a scenario might be unlikely, just knowing that it is possible helps to relieve the race shirt blues a little bit.

TEACH YOUR CHILDREN WELL

"Baseball's a great sport – but it's definitely not the most active game in town. It's a game of patience and strategy, of ritual and tradition, and of handing down lessons and memories from one generation to the next. We've both participated in this tradition, but we feel that running offers many of these same benefits that draw people to baseball."

"So give it a try, and take a child for a run sometime. Who knows? You might end up discovering a hidden athlete in an otherwise ordinary kid."

National Pastime

Springtime is finally upon us, which for many sports fans brings the familiar sounds of our national pastime: the crack of the bat (or the ping of aluminum), the smack of a pitch into the catcher's glove, and singing "Take Me Out to the Ballgame" while root, root, rooting for the home team.

Like clockwork, Little League practices have sprung up all over the place lately. Given the huge number of kids who play baseball, we often wonder about the relative fitness value for the children involved, especially when compared to our own favorite pastime of running.

Baseball's a great sport – but it's definitely not the most active game in town. It's a game of patience and strategy, of ritual and tradition, and of handing down lessons and memories from one generation to the next. We've both participated in this tradition, but we feel that running offers many of these same benefits that draw people to baseball.

It also shouldn't surprise you to learn that in some ways we prefer the sport of running over baseball, especially when we compare children's races to typical Little League gatherings.

We've all seen Little League games where kids in the field wander aimlessly, pull daisies in the outfield, scuff their shoes in the infield dirt, or yell out repeated choruses of "Hey batter, batter!" while chewing on their mitts. And those are the kids who are IN the game.

The kids in the dugout have lots of time to eat snacks or conduct clever contests like seeing who can blow the biggest bubble, or who can take off and put on their jacket the fastest. Clearly, it's not wall-to-wall action after the umpire shouts "Play Ball!"

Luckily, many of the kids who play baseball are generally athletic types who also enjoy playing catch in the backyard, or chasing after balls in the outfield during batting practice. Baseball players strive to maximize their skills and coordination, a process that succeeds only with constant repetition.

But what about kids who don't enjoy chattering in the infield, and dislike the taste of chewing on leather? There's no reason for kids to be inactive in the springtime simply because they don't like baseball. Even those who play Little League could still use a bit of extra physical activity.

That's where running (or any aerobic activity) comes in. As a matter of fact, you are probably better served by taking your kid on a 30-minute jog or bike ride a few times per week than spending that time shuttling them back and forth to practices and games. Your exercise time can double as family bonding time, and you can do it in any of the city parks or school playgrounds or wooded trails that your area has to offer.

Check your local area for 5K races or track meets during the spring and summer, especially if they have separate children's categories along with the main events. These are usually fun family activities where every child feels like a winner afterwards. They're also great opportunities to create traditions and memories with your kids that are just as strong as flipping through a game program in a crowded baseball stadium.

The catchphrase from *Field of Dreams* was, "If you build it, they will come." It's a great line from a great baseball movie – and we're going to steal it. Your local races have already been built by people who care about health and fitness and have a passion for running. All that's left is for you to come and enjoy them.

That way, you can make running and health your family's favorite pastime.

Donald Buraglio and Michael Dove

Just Run for Our Kids

Now that the school year is starting, we want to make sure your children have the opportunity to participate in Monterey County's Just Run program.

Just Run is a free program designed by running, fitness, and nutritional experts that is geared toward promoting fitness and healthy lifestyle choices in 2nd through 8th grade children. It provides a wealth of information for students, educators, and parents on starting and maintaining a fitness and nutritional program. Everyone knows about the problem of childhood obesity; programs like Just Run are part of the solution.

One aspect is called "Just Run Across the United States" where classes or youth groups cooperatively accumulate mileage in a virtual run across the United States, which is tracked on the website. Hundreds of locations are web-linked on this trip showing geographic, historical, nutritional, and otherwise interesting locations on the cross-country journey.

Last year, several classes from Carmel River School ran over 6,400 miles – enough mileage to run from Monterey to Boston and back to Monterey. Along the way they learned about the Native Americans of Skull Valley, Utah, studied the Mississippi River while crossing it, and passed the home of Punxsutawney Phil in Pennsylvania.

Individual incentive awards such as shirts, wrist bands, certificates, and plastic mileage tokens are provided to children who accumulate certain mileage totals while helping their class to run across the USA. But they only qualify for incentive awards if they also do "Just Deeds," or acts of good citizenship. In this way the program not only promotes fitness but responsible and honorable behavior.

Each school receives visits and training clinics from local elite runners. These athletes are excellent role models of fitness and health, and by running alongside the kids, they motivate our children to emulate them. They speak to the children about healthy eating, "Just Running Away" from drugs and smoking, and about helping their classmates succeed as well.

Children who run with their families receive double mileage in order to encourage family activity time. Running, walking, or rolling for those in wheelchairs all count toward mileage goals.

For more information about the Just Run program or how to institute it at your school, visit their website at www.justrun.org.

**Author's note: Monterey County's Just Run program guidelines are available to schools all over the country – see the website above for details.*

Birth of a Runner

"It wasn't as hard as I thought."

Those were my (Donald's) seven-year-old son's first words when I asked him about his race at the Big Sur 5K last weekend. It was his first ever 5K, and had you asked me four months ago whether he would ever enter a road race, I would have thought you were crazy.

He's never been an athletic kid, and he has never had any interest in playing organized sports. So you can imagine my surprise three months ago when he told me he wanted to sign up for the race.

He wasn't motivated by a desire to get in shape or to race against his schoolmates; he took a nobler, more selfless route to the starting line. As it turns out, the primary reason he wanted to enter was because he knew it was a fundraiser for his school.

The Big Sur Marathon board has a strong commitment to youth fitness programs, and the 5K was created specifically for local elementary and middle school students to participate with family members. The marathon gives financial awards to participating schools, in amounts based on the size of the school and the percentage of students who enter.

That was enough to hook my son, who has this innate desire to make a positive impact on the world (it probably comes from his mom). He helped organize a rummage sale for tsunami victims last year, and raised money for Hurricane Katrina relief. He's the self-appointed 3-R's (reduce, reuse, recycle) watchdog at our house, and cleaned trash from our neighborhood streets on Earth Day.

So when he learned that his participation might help his school, he was in. Never mind that he could barely run a lap without stopping or tripping over himself. The kid's a humanitarian.

We spent one day per week running laps around his schoolyard, taking walking breaks whenever he needed them. We gradually built up our distance, and the amount of time spent jogging instead of walking.

Eventually we expanded our horizons and explored some trails at a nearby county park that he hadn't seen before. He discovered new aspects of himself and the world around him that he didn't know about just a few months ago.

The time spent in shared activity helped us connect with each other, also. We talked about school and friends, and discussed whatever questions popped into his head during the course of our exercise time.

And by the time the Big Sur 5K rolled around, he was ready. He had no doubts about his ability to finish, because he and I had done all the proper preparation together. He was able to jog almost the whole distance with his Mom, and hit the post-race buffet with plenty of energy to spare. All in all, it was a great experience for him. He's even started asking about future races.

But here's the thing: I had no idea that this unathletic, noncompetitive kid would get hooked on any kind of sport, let alone one that happens to be my favorite. The fact that he ran a 5K with relative ease speaks volumes about the potential of children to make rapid improvements in their physical abilities.

Best of all, even if he doesn't ever race again, he's developed an excitement for running which will carry over into a generally healthier lifestyle. It's one of the most important benefits that the Big Sur Marathon gives to our community: promoting increased participation in healthy activity for children.

So give it a try, and take a child for a run sometime. Who knows? You might end up discovering a hidden athlete in an otherwise ordinary kid.

Fast Times at the Heart & Sole Races

Our (Donald's) family spent a recent Saturday morning in Salinas for the Heart & Sole Races. I was looking forward to the event for a couple of reasons:

1. My 7-year-old son wanted to try another 5K, this time with me accompanying him instead of his Mom, and...
2. My employer is the primary sponsor of the races, and it's never a bad idea to put in some face time at a company charity event. Plus, it's always amusing to see your flabby co-workers and supervisors walking around in running shorts.

Since I wasn't running the race competitively (well, sort of...you'll see), I thought I'd keep a diary of the events for a race report:

8:10AM: My son and I turn in our registration forms, and my friend Mike is working at the table. When my son is out of earshot, I lean over and half-jokingly ask Mike, "So how does the under-10 competition look?" OK, maybe it was one-quarter-jokingly. I'm pretty sure I was joking a little bit.

8:30: The Heart & Sole Race is underway! For all but two people, that is. My son was crossing and bending his legs throughout the National Anthem, and we finally headed over to the porta-potty just as the Star-Spangled Banner was yet waving; so much for getting a jump on the field.

8:31: My son exits the porta-potty, and our race is underway!

8:44: Mile 1 completed in 12:05. When we were training, the farthest the kid ran continuously was a single mile. So when I ask if he needs a walking break, and he shakes me off, I'm more than a little impressed. He's got his game face on.

8:50-8:55: We are slowly gaining on a young-looking boy running alongside his iPod-wearing mom. Without realizing it, I start accelerating to reel him in, leaving my son a few paces behind. I slow to my son's pace again, and nonchalantly say, "Hey, that boy looks about your age." No response; the kid is either focused or oblivious. Either way, we're still jogging.

8:56: Mile 2 completed, total time 24:00. Pace holding steady. We're still jogging. And we finally pass iPod mom and her kid.

9:05: A young-looking boy catches up and runs beside us for a while. Before he moves ahead of us, I give him an enthusiastic "Nice job, keep it up," followed a few seconds later by "So, how old are you, anyway?" You know … just trying to be friendly.

9:08: We see the finish line and my son hits the jets, as I look over my shoulder to see if any other kids are gaining on us. We're in the clear; I can relax now.

9:09: We cross the finish line in 37:14. For my son, this is a 6-minute PR over his time at the Big Sur 5K 3 weeks ago. At this rate, he'll be running sub-20 minutes by the end of the summer.

9:10: In the finisher's chute, a 40-something woman behind us tells my son, "You were my inspiration to keep going!" Apparently she had been only 5-10 yards behind us for the last two miles. This was her first 5K, and my 7-year-old kid helped her finish. How cool is that?

10:15: Heat 1 of the toddler trot features my 4-year-old daughter blasting away from the competition for a decisive victory. OK, there were only two other 4-year-old kids in the race, but still, my girl looked awesome. She'll move up an age division next year, but she's left behind a 4-and-under course record that could stand for years.

10:20: In Heat 3 of the toddler trot, my 2-year-old daughter jumps out to an early lead and gradually pulls away for another convincing win. With victories from both girls, I'm feeling like Venus and Serena Williams's father at the 2001 US Open when both daughters reached the final.

10:25: The buildup to the eagerly-awaited Salinas Valley Fruit and Vegetable Dash has all the odds-makers guessing. The carrot has the best runner's physique, but the chili pepper has been a bundle of energy all morning. The zucchini has a score to settle after everybody has mistakenly been calling her a cucumber all morning.

The race was hotly-contested, with contact among the runners and several lead changes to keep the crowd buzzing. The grape bunch surged at the line to win by a belly, just edging out the strawberry and the chili pepper. Results will become official after the grapes submit the obligatory urine sample and pass the drug screen.

10:30: Heading back to the car, I check the age group 5K results. My son was 5th in his 10-and-under age group, behind one ten-year-old, two nine-year-olds, and an eight-year-old. Not a bad showing for the kid – and he has three more years to conquer this division if he keeps at it.

10:40: Best aspect of the Heart & Sole: every kid in every race gets a medal. As our family walks back to the van, my kids are wearing medals (or, as my 4-year-old daughter predictably calls it, her "necklace") and talking about the good time they had. My wife and I tell them how proud we are of everybody, and they're all talking about doing it again next year.

The medals on these kids are merely an outward sign of what their parents already knew: they're all winners to us.

Donald Buraglio and Michael Dove

Dear Mrs. Obama

Dear Mrs. Obama,

Thank you for making the fight against youth obesity your primary concern as First Lady. As runners, parents, and community activists, we share your passion in this challenge.

We completely agree with the goals you have established: access to healthy, affordable food for all kids; increased physical activity in schools and in the community; healthier school meal programs; parents empowered with the information and tools to make good choices.

Since we have some experience in this area, we thought perhaps we could share some of our ideas and observations with you.

Make physical education and active recess mandatory from kindergarten to 12th grade: Include activities and lessons to emphasize how running or other aerobic exercise should become a lifetime habit. This is a low-cost initiative, needing no equipment and no new teachers: for example, Monterey County's Just Run program is free, can be led by any teacher or parent, and has positively impacted more than 7,500 kids.

Health education should be an important part of school rather than an afterthought. Having "No child left inside" is just as important as "No child left behind."

Make BMI measurements and fitness goals part of school programs: This might be a controversial step – but any executive will tell you that you can't manage what you can't measure. Kids should know their fitness levels – and these assessments are a great way to open a dialogue with parents as well.

Simplify: Please avoid the typical bureaucratic solution of just throwing more money and researchers at the problem. We all know that poor nutrition + sedentary lifestyle = obesity. Most health agencies already have programs in place – the problem is that those programs haven't been working. Find the few good programs out there (see Just Run above) to direct resources toward, and make them more accessible nationwide.

Use "foot soldiers": Any battle needs lots of foot soldiers. In this case, use established community organizers and advocates, and recruit new ones as well. Newly proposed programs should have advocates in every school, workplace, and health organization. Encourage people to get involved at school or in the community.

Lose the anti-running bias: Maybe we're paranoid, but we'll put this one out there ... we're a bit offended that the Surgeon General's *Vision for a Healthy and Fit Nation 2010* says children should have 60 minutes a day of vigorous exercise but doesn't mention running. Included in the activity examples are softball, racquetball, kayaking (Really? In inner cities?), skating, mall walking, and washing the car, but somehow running didn't make the list.

The President's Active Lifestyle award is based on kids being active 5 days a week for 6 weeks. 100 activities are mentioned and running is (thankfully) one of them, but so are archery, billiards, croquet, darts, gardening, horseshoe pitching, ski-mobiling, skeet shooting, and even shuffleboard.

See, here's the thing: running is the simplest, cheapest, most accessible and most effective means of exercise there is. Although we risk offending the kayaking or shuffleboard lobbies by saying this, we feel our sport deserves a much higher profile in fitness programs.

Make it permanent: Kids need more than 6 total weeks of exercise; it has to be daily, it has to be a life-long habit, and it has to be fun and rewarding in order to be successful. If your legacy is a generation of healthy, happy kids, that's something to be enormously proud of.

Good luck with your initiative, and feel free to contact us if you need some free consulting!

A FEW ROAD HAZARDS

"Many avid runners become so hooked on the sport that it often consumes their thoughts. Sure, a hardcore runner may appear alert and attentive on the surface – but it's a good bet that internally, that otherwise normal-appearing person is completely preoccupied with all manner of details pertaining to his or her running."

"All runners engage in a sort of internal decision-making process to answer that question. Like everything else in life, running comes with its share of risks. The question we all answer is whether the benefits we get from running and racing outweigh the potential risk."

The Injury Life

We typically utilize this column space to describe all of the benefits of running – however, sometimes it might be possible to have too much of a good thing.

Many avid runners become so hooked on the sport that it often consumes their thoughts. Sure, a hardcore runner may appear alert and attentive on the surface – but it's a good bet that internally, that otherwise normal-appearing person is completely preoccupied with all manner of details pertaining to his or her running.

He (or she) will spend countless waking hours thinking about how many miles he logged that day, what his average time for the run was, when and where his next run will be, how many total miles he's run this week, how much longer it will be until he needs a new pair of shoes, which running clothes he needs to buy once the weather changes, how much fluid he should be consuming during the day, when his next race is going to be, and whether one of those nagging sore areas is going to turn into an injury.

That last point is a critical one – because when a runner develops physical problems, all other concerns get pushed to the back burner. Runners are notorious for having tunnel vision when it comes to focusing on (and worrying about) anything that prevents them from doing the activity they love. Unfortunately, injuries are an all too common occurrence among this crowd.

For example, here's a typical conversation that might take place between any of our group of friends who cross paths in their everyday (non-running) lives. Let's say they meet unexpectedly on Main Street this week. They certainly have a wide variety of discussion topics to mull over: the economy, the upcoming election, the war, career changes, or family developments. Despite all of that, it's a virtual certainty that the conversation would unfold something like this:

Joe: "Hi Susie, haven't seen you for awhile. How are you doing?"

Susie: "Good to see you, Joe. I'm OK but I've hardly been running at all. My piriformis problem just isn't going away. I've been stretching, doing ice massage, and taking Advil. I'm even going to Bikram yoga a few times a week, which helps for a few hours, but by the next morning it's bothering me again."

Joe: "That's too bad. I haven't been running much either. My left shin is really painful when I run, and hurts all day long afterward. I had an x-ray and MRI last week and there's no stress fracture right now, but the doc says it looks imminent if I keep running. I don't think it's shin splints. It could be compartment syndrome. I'm seeing my physical therapist but the progress seems really slow. Occasionally I'll try the elliptical machine but it gets too boring after a while."

Susie: "Yeah. It's really frustrating … Oh, look, there's Ted."

Ted: "What a coincidence. How are you guys? Sorry I haven't made the group runs lately - I've been decreasing my mileage because of some Achilles tendonitis. Luckily it's not a complete tear, but when I run it's extremely painful. I'm also doing some pool running, but I don't get the same endorphin high in the water. And I feel like everyone's laughing at me when I'm wearing my swim suit."

Joe: "Yeah, I hate it when that happens. My wife just had a knee operation for patellofemoral syndrome and did some pool running during her rehab. She's favoring her right side a bit now, so her left plantar fascia is becoming a problem. She does ice massage and flexion exercises using toe curls and a towel. It takes about an hour a day – really a hassle."

Ted: "Hey Susie … how is Dave doing?"

Susie: "He hasn't been running a lot either. His right hip hurts and he aggravated his left illiotibial band because he was running strangely to protect his hip. He's going to both the physical therapist and chiropractor but still has problems. He's also trying myofascial release therapy and it seems to be helping a little."

Ted: "Wow, good luck to him for sure. Did you hear about Rod? He ran a race last month and right near the end he pulled a calf muscle. He had to beat someone in his age group so he gutted it out, but now he's injured again. He's doing intermittent heat and ice treatments. He also sees a massage therapist twice a week for deep muscle work. Hope he gets better soon."

Joe: "So … are we all running at the regular place tomorrow morning? 12 miles on the rec trail starting at 5AM?"

Susie: "Sounds great to me. See you then."

Ted: "Someone should call Rod and tell him – he'll probably show up."

Joe: "Yeah. It will be great to talk with everyone again!"

Running Annoyances

Sometimes, in the interest of journalistic integrity, a minor sports story might be dismissed by professional writers in favor of something more meaningful. However, for amateur hacks like the two of us, no topic is too trivial for our column space.

That's how we noticed a recent story about "spin class rage," and considered the potential for something similar to happen within our local running community. But first, some background:

Last month, a Wall Street stock broker was charged with assault after he became enraged during a cycling class at a posh Manhattan health club. During his high-intensity spin class, he apparently became so fed up by a fellow club member's grunting and moaning, that he shoved the offender off his bike and slammed him into a wall.

The attorney for the grunter called the attack "spin rage," and filed a criminal complaint charging that the attack caused a back injury to his client. He maintains that the grunter was merely enjoying the "euphoric experience" of cycling, and making noises to increase his endorphin high.

This isn't merely some urban legend we've crafted; do you think we could make a story like that up? However, it did get us to thinking about what kinds of runners might send us over the edge someday during the midst of a routine Saturday 12-miler through Pebble Beach.

In other words ... is there a possibility of hearing about a "run rage" attack someday? And if so, what kind of runner would trigger such an outburst?

Honestly, it wouldn't be a situation like the case in New York. Grunting is somewhat commonplace among a group of hard-working runners – especially during a difficult track workout. And if we were intolerant of moaning, we'd have clobbered one or two friends of ours many years ago.

But we can certainly think of plenty of runner behaviors that are annoying – so many, in fact, that we've assembled a list below.

However, before getting to the list, we need to emphasize that we would NEVER condone a "run rage" reaction to anybody. On the other hand, if you recognize yourself in any of these descriptions, be on notice that you may be bugging the heck out of your training partners.

One other note worth mentioning is that we're using "guy" most frequently here, because guys are the most common offenders - but you can use "guy" or "girl" interchangeably for virtually all of these. Here then, is our list of the most likely targets of "run annoyance":

- The guy who shows up just as the group is leaving, then asks everyone to wait while he puts his shoes on.
- The guy who says it's going to be an "easy day," then takes off at 6-minute mile pace.
- The guy who launches a snot rocket without looking, and nails your ankle while you're beside him.

- The guy who complains about how terrible his training is going, even though he's running more mileage or more days per week than you.
- The girl wearing an iPod who doesn't hear you say, "On your left!" as you're passing, then drifts over and collides with you, and freaks out because you startled her.
- The guy who tells the same story or joke he's already told several times on previous runs.
- The guy who has to wait up for you at the top of a big climb, then tells you how his injuries are bothering him today.
- The stats nerd who knows the on-base percentage and slugging percentages of every player on the Giants and A's, and wants to make sure you know them too by the end of the run.
- The guy wearing the GPS who announces every tenth of a mile.
- The girl not wearing a GPS who keeps asking "How far have we gone now?"
- The guy who keeps telling you how fast he was 10 years ago, or how the training group where he used to live had all kinds of great runners.
- The guy who pulls off to the side for a "pit stop," but does his business in plain sight because he's too lazy to move completely off the road or trail.
- The walkers who won't move from in lanes 1 and 2 of the track while a group of runners are trying to run interval workouts.
- The guy who speeds up when he hears another runner behind him, to avoid being passed – especially when he learns the other runner is a girl.
- The middle-aged guy in a race who puts on a furious sprint to outlean some little kid at the tape so he can finish in 642nd place instead of 643rd.
- The girl who goes on and on about all the problems associated with her "cycle" while running with a group of guys.
- The guy who speeds up to run in front of you, then breaks wind a few seconds later.

- The guy who blows his nose into his palm while running, then goes around shaking everyone's hand after the run.
- The guy who never carries fluids, but always asks for a drink from your bottle during long runs.
- The sweaty, smelly guy who tries to chat up every cute girl running on the rec trail.

Do any of these items sound like anyone you know? More importantly, do they sound like YOU? If so, let this be a word of caution for you: other runners notice these things. And they don't like them. So for all of our sakes, please try to refrain from anything on the list above.

After all, the euphoric experience of running isn't justification to irritate the heck out of people.

Calculated Risks

"If you knew there was a possibility that something terrible might someday happen, would you stop doing something you loved?"

That question popped into our inbox late in 2008, shortly after marathons made front page news for the worst possible reason: the deaths of competitors at separate events in October and November. Honestly, we're still not sure what the correct answer should be.

In October, a 35-year-old man collapsed and died during the Chicago Marathon on a day of record heat and humidity in the Midwest. Four weeks later, elite runner Ryan Shay, extremely fit and only 28 years old, suffered heart failure while competing in the U.S. Olympic Marathon Trials. He collapsed after completing only five miles, and efforts to revive him were unsuccessful.

Shockwaves from Ryan Shay's death spread immediately through the running community, and was a topic of conversation for weeks afterward. Although the autopsy was inconclusive, Shay's father said Ryan was diagnosed with an enlarged heart at age 14 - yet he kept on running and racing. It was who he was.

Sadly, deaths in marathons are not unheard of, and shorter distance races also see their share of tragedy. Furthermore, such events appear unrelated to geographic location or to the victim's level of fitness. Our local community has even been impacted; two runners have died in the 22-year history of the Big Sur Marathon, and one runner suffered cardiac arrest and was revived during a 5K in Salinas this year.

Runner deaths like these are the shark attack stories of the endurance sports community: although they are exceedingly rare, they absolutely (and justifiably) terrify everybody to the point of rethinking their rationale for doing the activity in the first place. That was the implied basis of the question in our inbox: Is running dangerous? And if so, why do we continue to do it? Why do we push our bodies to extremes of performance that could someday prove fatal?

Every runner engages in a sort of internal decision-making process to answer that question. Like everything else in life, running comes with its share of risks. The question we all answer is whether the benefits we get from running and racing outweigh the potential risk.

With any activity, if the risk/benefit ratio is favorable, the activity appears acceptable. However, all of us have various definitions of "favorable" - a point that helps to explain sports such as BASE jumping or bull riding - which causes reasonable people to disagree about recommending certain activities.

People might tell us that runners have died in marathons. We'll reply that nearly all of those people – as was the case in October and November – had preexisting heart conditions that were either undiagnosed or untreated. There is a good chance that those individuals might have died very early deaths even if they were sedentary.

Others might say we're risking death by competing in marathons. We'd respond that our odds of dying in a car accident are about 200 times greater, but that doesn't stop us from driving. In fact, the odds of death in a person's lifetime are 6 times greater that you will drown in the bathtub, or 10 times greater that you'll perish from a fall out of your own bed. Everything is risky.

Some may recommend that we take up another activity – but to us, that is simply non-negotiable. The physical, emotional, and spiritual benefits we gain from running are far more than we are willing to give up for a vague suggestion of greater security.

We realize that to some people, that might sound reckless – and that's why there's no correct answer to the question posed at the top of the column. The two of us consider the risk of running to be incredibly small. However, if a cardiologist told us that we had a heart condition that could kill us if we continued to run, perhaps our answer would be different … but the decision would be a lot harder than you'd think. As country star Garth Brooks sings, "Yes, my life is better left to chance/ I could have missed the pain but I'd of had to miss the dance."

All we know for sure, above all else, is how thankful we are for the gifts that running has provided us. We're thankful for the ability to do the activities we love, to whatever degree we desire, in the beautiful surroundings that we're lucky enough to call home.

We also understand that nothing is promised, and there's a slight possibility that each day's run could be our last. However, if it were all taken away tomorrow, we still wouldn't do it any other way. We've each been fortunate to experience so many wonderful things from running and racing, that we would still be forever grateful.

So today, we're giving thanks for the sport that means so much to us, for the opportunities and experiences it has provided, and for all of the miles in life we've covered so far. We can only hope that we'll continue to be blessed with many more in the future.

OFF TO THE RACES!

"Western States took me to some unbelievable places, both physically and psychologically. Some were wondrous and exciting. Others were dark and terrifying. A few were just plain bizarre. The end result was a journey that was both humbling and empowering, discouraging yet ultimately uplifting."

"Here's the good part: our gain for suffering through all of this is something akin to enlightenment. We understand that our bodies and minds are capable of far more than most people ever realize; that the primary limiting factors in life's journeys are the extent to which our minds can dream, and to which we're willing to work to achieve them."

Three Minutes at the Top of the Stairs

Approximately 500 vertical feet below the 14,115' summit of Pikes Peak stands a sign that says "16 Golden Stairs" – which is both a welcome and foreboding sight for weary runners.

The term refers to the final 32 switchbacks (a stair is one pair of switchbacks) before reaching the summit. Fred Barr, the main developer of the trail that bears his name, chose the Biblical allusion for this final, steepest portion of the ascent, symbolizing a golden stairway that climbs to heaven.

After climbing for over 3 hours and 7300' to reach the signpost, I (Donald) faced about 20 more minutes of struggle before reaching the summit that is the turnaround point of the Pikes Peak Marathon.

Every course description I read in preparation for the race gave similar advice about what to do after reaching the summit: get out of there fast. Spend as little time in the thin air as possible, so your body doesn't become too oxygen-starved for the second half of the run. Get your bib marked, fill your water bottle, and start quickly back down the mountain.

But I had trained for too long, traveled too far, and worked too hard in the race to reach this point; I couldn't simply turn and leave the summit behind without taking its proper measure. So after clicking my watch at 3 hours, 40 minutes, I moved off to one side and stood quietly, taking in as much of the scene as my aching, dizzy, lethargic brain could absorb.

For some people, the vantage point of tremendous height opens the mind and stimulates creative passion. Ancient philosophers and gifted artists have wiled away hours atop high mountains, seeking inspiration or enlightenment. Songwriter Katharine Bates wrote the lyrics to "America the Beautiful" on the summit of Pikes Peak, probably very close to the spot upon which I now stood.

From this perspective, it was easy to see that God did indeed shed His grace on this majestic purple mountain. The splendor all around me was overwhelming, and I gazed in awe of the surroundings, whispering the word "beautiful" more times than I can remember.

In typical fashion, as I contemplated all of these lofty ideas, my thoughts eventually turned more inward and introspective. I couldn't help but ponder all of the gifts in my life that helped me reach this point.

I have been blessed with a body that is capable of running (well, mostly running ... I needed some walking breaks) up the grueling trail, despite my frequent neglect of its basic needs like good nutrition and adequate rest. I thought of my wife, and all of the years she has patiently supported my obsession with running, and my constant pursuit of newer, more time-consuming challenges. I pictured my young children, hoped for a day when they can feel the happiness and satisfaction I felt at that moment, and wishing there was some way I could capture a small measure of this experience for their limited comprehension. I thought of all of my training partners who have encouraged me as I prepared for this day.

I concluded that there is great beauty to be found within my own life, comparable to the natural beauty of the mountain, but more intimate. It was there with me all along my journey, and burst into the open like a song at the top of the hill.

The summit of Pikes Peak is possibly the closest I'll ever come to glimpsing heaven while standing on Earth. Before leaving, I vowed that I would have to return there someday, lest the vision ever diminishes. I filled my water bottle, asked a volunteer to take my picture, and picked up two rocks to carry down the hill with me - one for each of my kids' rock collections. I clicked my watch, noted the elapsed time - 2 minutes, 48 seconds - and started my long descent of the mountain.

Despite the thin air, despite the increasing pain in my legs and feet, and despite the creeping exhaustion of mind and body, I smiled nearly all the way down.

Donald Buraglio and Michael Dove

Let's Put on a Race

Lately we have been discouraged about the passing of several local races; we counted up all the former events we've seen come and go, and came up with nearly 30 of them over the past 20 years. So why is it so hard to maintain a road race, anyway?

For the answer, let's eavesdrop on the town council of Pancake Flats, as they discuss putting on a local 5K. Maybe we'll learn a bit about race economics and politics. The Mayor is presiding.

* * *

Ms. Mayor: "Let's schedule the 5K for the first Sunday in May in order to show off our city, bring in tourists, and get our families fit and healthy. Let's try to get 300 runners."

Minister Brown: "But Ms. Mayor, Sunday is the Lord's Day. We don't want people staying away from church."

Ms. Mayor: "Can we do Saturday then, Rabbi Ginsburg?"

Rabbi: "Vell, I von't run … but it vill be OK, ve'll suffer through it."

Ms. Mayor: "I thought we'd start at the town square and run south on 2nd Street and turn around and come back."

Mrs. Smith: "Then no one will see our businesses on the north side of town! Let's start at Northside Mall and run to the Town Square instead."

Ms. Mayor: "If we do that, we'll need buses to take people back to the start area when the race is over. I'm sure the school district or the transit company will donate them for such a fine cause."

Mrs. Williams (Head of the School Board) and Mr. Richards (President of the transit company) both speak at the same time: "Hey – times are tough, budgets are restricted, gas is prohibitive, insurance is expensive, we have to pay overtime on Saturday, and you'll need 8 buses and drivers and the minimum rental is 4 hours. The best we can do – and this is a bargain – is $6,500."

Mr. Randazzo (head of the Town Council): "While we're talking about money, even though this is a city event, you need to pay the City's event fee of $500 and the use fee for the Town Square of $500."

Mr. Badge (Chief of Police): "For all those road closures, we'll need a dozen officers for overtime on Saturday to handle traffic control. That will be $2,000. And don't forget you've got to close the freeway offramps at 2nd Street, so you'll need State Dept. of Transportation permits for $500."

Mr. Clean (Chief of Sanitation): "Make sure we have enough Porta-Potties. They're $50 each and $100 for the disabled ones. You can never have too many Porta-Potties, so I'll provide 10 at the start and 10 at the end and 3 at each of your three aid stations. Oh, and don't forget about cleanup at the end. That will be about $2,000."

Ms. Mayor: "Why do we need disabled Porta-Potties at a race?"

Mr. Clean: "It's state law, and for spectators, and you might have some wheelchair participants. And I almost forgot – we want a green race don't we? That costs another $750."

Ms. Mayor: "Green race?! What makes our race green?"

Mr. Clean: "We leave no environmental footprint. Just let me worry about that. That's what you pay me for."

Mr. Fabrizzi (union representative): "I'll make you a deal – we'll charge you rock bottom for setting up the tables and awards stands and everything you need at the finish line. I can get my guys for $3,000. Set up, take down. No worries."

Ms. Mayor: "This is getting out of hand. Why can't we just have some volunteers set up the tables?"

Mr. Fabrizzi: "It's a union town - that's how you got elected, Ms. Mayor. And no one sets up an event in this town without union workers."

Ms. Mayor: "How about you Mrs. Smith – you're the Pancake Flats running club President. What do the runners want?"

Mrs. Smith: "We expect the Pancake Flats 5K to have all the usual amenities of other races. The course needs to be USATF certified ($1,800) and sanctioned ($300). We want long sleeve technical-fabric shirts for all participants ($4,500), and finishers medals for everyone ($1100). Awards 5 deep in each 5 year age group for both men and women from under 15 to 85 and over ($3,000) are standard. We need large, highly visible mile markers ($1,000). Rock bands at each mile and at the finish area ($2,500) would be great. We also need chip timing and timing mats at each mile so we can see our splits on the Internet the next day. ($10,000). That's about it."

Ms. Mayor: "Is that ALL?"

Mrs. Smith: "Well, that's not counting food – coffee at the start, and a buffet at the finish. Not just the usual bananas, Gatorade, and energy bars – but maybe free beer, bratwurst, pancakes, or sandwiches ($3000). Great food gets you a lot more runners for sure. "

Ms Mayor: "And I'd like to ask the City Attorney, Mr. Counsel, what do you think?"

Mr. Counsel: "We need race liability. I'd say about $1,000 for race day insurance. Don't forget medical support and two ambulances and doctors on duty just in case anything happens ($3,000). And we need communication systems to make sure this all works ($2,500)."

Ms. Mayor: "Wow. Is there anything I've forgotten?"

Mrs. Smith: "We haven't mentioned basic race expenses: advertising ($1,000), race bibs ($200), printing of race brochures and entry blanks ($1,500), creating and managing a race website ($1,500), start and finish banners and traffic control signage ($3,000). Most races collect money for charity as well, maybe $5,000 donated to some local causes."

Ms. Mayor: "I'd like to ask Mr. Balance, our City Treasurer, based on our discussion today to compute what our race entry fee would be to break even."

Mr. Balance: "Well, we have around $70,000 in expenses and I'm sure we've forgotten some so let's round it to $75,000. We're expecting 300 runners, so we'll have to charge $250 for our 5K in order to break even."

Mrs. Smith: "That's CRAZY. No runners will show up at that price. The city of Rolling Hills has a 5K that's only $25."

Ms. Mayor: "Yes, but our Pancake Flats will be the BEST 5K EVER!"

* * *

And chances are, it won't be around for the following year.

Where Everybody Knows My Name

The Los Angeles Marathon likes to be innovative. They were the first West Coast marathon to use the now-ubiquitous space blankets we see after every race. They were also the first major marathon to use chip timing for more accurate results, which render bib numbers unnecessary except for their nostalgic appeal.

This year the marathon capitalized on that needlessness by attempting to start another new trend in racing: placing the participant's name on their bib, in addition to a traditional race number. Anyone who pre-registered for the race by a set deadline had this new feature automatically provided for him or her.

At first glance, I (Donald) figured this was some kind of corny gimmick, in a city that is known for creating a lot of them - the marathon equivalent of *Joe Millionaire*. The idea also made me a bit apprehensive in a Big Brother sort of way; at most races, I tend to be a quiet observer, taking in the scene around me, but keeping to myself and enjoying the experience in a somewhat introspective manner. Even though I'm sharing the day with thousands of people, I generally prefer to be anonymous.

On race morning in Los Angeles, I quickly found out that things would be different.

It began as I stood in silence in the parking garage elevator, staring down at my feet, and suddenly heard a cheerful voice say, "Well, are you ready, Donald?" It took me a second to wonder how this complete stranger knew my name, and then I remembered. So I told Hiroshi that I felt OK, wished him luck, and resigned myself to commencing a weird day.

A few other people greeted me by name, and I reciprocated. In a strange way, I felt like I didn't have a choice; I kept having flashbacks to the *Seinfeld* episode where people posted their names and photos by the elevator, became uncomfortably friendly with each other, then turned resentful and angry with anyone who didn't follow the new code of openness and camaraderie. The last thing I needed was to irritate an anxious mob of runners.

As the race unfolded, I began to suspend my early judgment of having my name on my bib, and the gimmick became more of a curiosity to me. Part of the intrigue was wondering what name the spectators would yell; although I signed up for the race under my proper name, many folks shortened it like we were longtime friends. Others tried to cover their bases by yelling multiple versions like "Go Donald! All right Donny! Go Don! Go D!"

My name also changed depending on what area of town we were in. Most of the Mexican spectators called me "Donaldo", and periodically I heard the incessant LA Marathon cheer of *Si, se puede!* replaced by *Andale, Donaldo!* In Koreatown the locals got tripped up by that pesky l/r thing, and my name often came out as "Do-nard" - but they said it with such enthusiasm that it still felt good to hear.

Complete strangers expressed a sometimes frightening level of good spirit towards me. Somewhere on Exposition Blvd, an enormous woman with a booming voice stood on the street corner and shouted "WHOOOOO! Yeaaah, Donny baby! You looking GOOD to me! I'd like to eat you up!" I picked up my pace around that particular turn, more out of nervousness than inspiration, but it did help move me down the road.

At each aid station it seemed as if the volunteers had been waiting just for me to arrive. They handed out cups and said things like, "Here you go, Donald!" and as I thanked them for the cup, I heard, "You're welcome, Donald!" in reply. The thought crossed my mind that maybe next year the volunteers could wear name bibs, too - that way, runners could call out "I want YOUR cup, Eddie!" or, "Nice handoff, Maria!" Friendships could be forged in the passing of Gatorade cups. I've certainly met people in stranger ways.

I became entertained by hearing my name in ways I never had before. On one corner, a punk-rock band hammered out some rapid-fire one-chord song, with the singer growling "run, run, run, run" into the microphone, interspersed with people's names he saw, including mine. The Crenshaw High cheerleaders put my name into a cheer while they were jumping and kicking on the sidewalk. Late in the race, I passed a Spanish radio broadcaster's booth, and I'm pretty sure I heard my name mentioned by the commentator. Unfortunately, it was in the same sentence as the words *despacio* (slow) and *lucha* (struggle) - but hey, sometimes it feels good just to be noticed.

By the time the race was over, I had changed my mind about the whole name-wearing thing. There aren't many ways to make a race of over 20,000 people feel intimate and personal, but this is certainly one of them. It definitely made the race more memorable, almost entirely for the better.

At this point, there's no telling if the L.A. experiment will last. Now that the novelty is faded, I'm sure plenty of people will take advantage of the system to create trash-talk names *a la* the XFL, or try to sneak dirty names past the race censors like they do with license plates at the DMV. There's no shortage of people willing to ruin a good idea. Then again, this may turn out to be the wave of the future.

I'm sure that in most of my future races I'll go back to the same reticent, inconspicuous person I usually am. But the next time I enter the L.A. Marathon, I'll know that all the course is a stage, and everyone is a player. I'll gladly reprise my role as Donald the Runner, and revel in my three hours of fame.

Donald Buraglio and Michael Dove

The Dipsea Race

Run around the trails of Northern California long enough, and you're sure to hear about the Dipsea Race, a world-famous 7.1-mile trail run through the hills of Marin County, from Mill Valley to Stinson Beach.

The Dipsea is truly a legendary race, held in almost religious regard amongst Bay Area trail runners. It is the second oldest footrace in the country (behind only the Boston Marathon), and this June will mark the 96th running. The motto of the Dipsea is "The Greatest Race", and it is definitely the most exciting event most people will ever run.

This race is not for the faint of heart. Although only slightly longer than a 10K, more than 75% of the race is on challenging single-track trail or fire roads. The course profile is simple: climb 650 feet, immediately descend 500', climb another 1360', then race downhill through the forest until you reach sea level at the beach.

It all starts in the picturesque town square of Mill Valley, but immediately turns nasty as runners ascend more than 670 stairs, the height equivalent of a fifty-story building, in order to reach the start of the trail. They cross Panoramic Highway, descend into Muir Woods National Monument, then start the second climb up and over Mount Tamalpais. The long final downhill includes railroad-tie stairs, river crossings, and jumping over an unmarked fencepost about a half-mile from the finish.

Different stretches of the course have distinctively intimidating names such as Cardiac, Steep Ravine, The Swoop, Insult Hill, and Dynamite. The most ominous name of all comes relatively early in the race. At a fork in the trail about 1.75 miles into the race, a sign is posted: one arrow on the sign points to a trail marked "Suicide", and the other arrow says "safer." As the race brochure will tell you, Suicide is the traditional racer's route.

The trail becomes crowded in many places, and hot weather causes dusty conditions which limit visibility and make footing very treacherous. Passing becomes dangerous on the long narrow stretches, especially if a competitor doesn't want to cede the trail. In these situations, the race turns into a full-contact sport, and it's not unusual to see people knocked to the ground. A good deal of time is also spent jumping over fallen runners who have tripped on precarious roots and rocks, or slipped on the steep slopes. Some runners even start the race wearing protective equipment that may become necessary deep in the forest.

The race is unique for several reasons. Foremost is its handicap-start system, which gives head start minutes based on gender and age. Thus, the oldest women and youngest kids leave first. Each minute thereafter, the other runners leave in groups according to their assigned handicap. By the time the 20- to 30-year-old men leave, the first runners have more than a 20-minute head start.

The handicap system streamlines the amount of runners on the single-track at any one time. It also means that younger, faster runners are constantly passing all those who started ahead of them. It's a game of survival that makes people irrational; for this one hour each year, I feel absolutely no shame about barging past old men or young girls as I'm storming through the trail. (Don't hate the player, hate the game.)

The first person to cross the finish line wins, and the only thing that matters is overall place; no age group or gender awards are given. The assigned handicap times are adjusted periodically to make the race more competitive. Typically the first five finishers include a combination of high-school runners, top 50- or 60-year-old age-groupers, or extremely fast open runners.

If you finish in the top 100 your place will be on your bib number the following year. The first 35 finishers are awarded a black shirt numbered with their overall finishing place. These shirts are coveted status symbols in Marin County, and are the most prized possession of any runner's collection - far more valuable than any PR or age group award.

Another unique aspect of the race is the "open course" system. Basically, once you leave Mill Valley, you're free to take any shortcuts through the forest that you know about. This provides a huge potential advantage to Marin County runners who frequently train on the Dipsea trail and explore various options to shave a few seconds wherever possible.

There are several places where the trail splits into branches, which reconnect at a later point. There is strategy involved with taking a longer, wider route instead of a more direct single-track which may be crowded. The consensus "best route" is marked, but racers are always dashing off through the woods at unmarked areas. However, it's risky to follow someone off the course, because there's no positive way of knowing if a "shortcut" is actually a faster route, or if you'll both end up getting lost or injured.

The race started as a 2-person contest in 1904, then grew into an invitational event, and eventually became open to the public. Entry into the race is somewhat complicated and intentionally favors Marin County runners. In order to limit damage to the trail, the race is limited to less than 1500 runners, although about 4000 apply. However, with persistence (and a good bribe- I'm not kidding), it is possible to obtain an entry.

I (Donald) love this race and fear it in almost equal amounts. Through the years, it has come to occupy a special place in my heart – and as race day draws near again, my heart beats a bit faster just thinking about it.

Dipsea by the Numbers

If you know anything about the world-famous Dipsea Race in Marin County, you understand that a single number means everything. Not the clock time, not your age group place – it's your overall finishing place that matters more than anything else.

Accordingly, my (Donald's) race report from this year's Dipsea will be strictly by the numbers:

96: Number of times, including this year, the Dipsea has been run – which is confusing, because last year was the 100th anniversary. But like the Boston Marathon and so many other sporting events, the Dipsea went on hiatus during the World War years. Could any of us imagine something like that happening today – a whole baseball season being called off, or the most popular recreational sporting events suspended for several years at a time? I mean … there's a war going on right now, isn't there? For various reasons, we don't make nearly the sacrifices our forbearers did in supporting our war efforts. In the grand scheme of things, that's probably not a good thing.

(Sorry, I didn't intend to turn this into "Meet the Press." Back to the running…)

22: Number of head start minutes the first runners had before I started the race. There are a lot of ways this race kicks you in the teeth, but I'll say this: there's no other event that rewards getting older quite so generously.

1: Number of head start minutes I receive. Apparently in the eyes of the Dipsea committee, I'm not very old yet.

3: Number of years I have to wait until I get another head start minute. You know, patience has never been one of my better qualities. I'm not sure how I'm going to get myself through the next 1094 days. Not that I'm counting.

8: Bib number on the guy next to me on the start line, meaning he came in 8th place last year. I exercised some prudence and took a couple of steps backwards so I wouldn't feel so discouraged when he left me in the dust. It was a humble but smart move.

2: Minutes at the beginning of the race where I felt completely terrified. I've already called this race intimidating, but that doesn't really do justice to the feeling of dread I have every year when taking off from the start – knowing the pain that lies ahead, and knowing that if I take the easy way out and run conservatively, I'll feel like a failure. I get so anxious during the first quarter mile that I almost feel like throwing up. Thankfully, after I hit the stairs, I'm usually able to find a rhythm and settle down a bit - but those first two minutes are always horribly gut-wrenching. I can't overemphasize this.

676: Number of stairs climbed in the first mile of the race. There's no better way to describe these stairs than as absolute quad killers. The Dipsea stairs are the signature challenge of this race, but after several decades of use, many of them have fallen into disrepair. This year the race committee started a fundraising drive to reconstruct portions of the stairs, to ensure that they inflict the same misery on generations of Dipsea runners to come.

1000: Number of dollars required to "sponsor" one of the new stairs. A plaque engraved with your name will be mounted on one of the Dipsea stairs for everybody to see. But here's the thing: these stairs already own me. So placing my name on one of them would make me feel like the girl who has her boyfriend's name tattooed on her backside. It's not exactly something I would want to be made public ... but maybe that's just me.

4: Number of kids knocked over by me during my 7.1 mile romp to Stinson Beach. For the record, two of them jumped in front of me unexpectedly when I was passing them, so they had what was coming to them. Although they all lost their footing, none of the kids actually hit the ground, at least from what I could tell. I'm sure they'll be fine. I prefer to think of the whole situation as me helping them build character. Because that's me: I'm all about the kids.

11: Age of the girl I found myself sprinting against during the final 200 meters. With about 100 meters to go, I was finally able to drop the hammer on her, and I didn't feel the least bit of shame in dropping her. Don't feel bad for the girl, though - at least I didn't have to knock her down to move past.

90: Minutes my friend Mike drove to see me at the finish line. He and his wife were staying in San Francisco for the weekend, and decided to come see the race I keep badgering him to enter. It was great to see him. I typically run this race by myself and don't know anybody at the finish area, so it felt nice to see a friendly face.

Despite my constant pleading, Mike doesn't have any interest in doing the Dipsea. In fact, seeing countless finishers cross the line muddy, limping and bloodied probably sealed the deal for him. But he came to see me anyway. Now that's a friend.

62: Age of the oldest man to run faster than me. Last year there was a 68-year-old who beat me, so I appear to be closing the gap on the sexagenarian men. As for the women...

52: Age of the oldest woman to beat me. One year ago I noticed this same 51-year-old who completely thrashed me – and she was back again this year. I'm not making any progress here.

Actually, I shouldn't even be writing about this age thing; it's such a no-win situation. Even if I get faster over the next few years and catch up to some of these 50- and 60-year-olds, I'll still get myself all tied up in knots worried about...

14: Age of youngest male and female runners to beat me. A girl ran the course two minutes faster, and a boy ran five minutes faster than me. This race attracts some amazing runners on both ends of the age spectrum.

10: Minutes between phone calls to my wife (at home in Carmel Valley) from Mike's cell phone as he drove me back to the start line after the race. The cell phone got poor reception amidst the tall redwoods and frequently cut out on us - which wouldn't have been so bad, except that Mike decided to start the conversation with a joke:

My wife: Hello?

Mike: Hey, it's Mike. Your husband's in the car with me. He's lying in the back seat, bleeding and almost passed out.

My wife: What? Really?

And that's when the cell phone reception died.

25: Approximate number in the batch of cherry chocolate chunk cookies, baked by my wife, that awaited me when I returned home. I'm fairly sure she had made them even before she thought I might be dying. My wife is pretty much a saint in the things she does for me and the nonsense she puts up with on a daily basis. It's occurred to me lately that I probably don't say that enough.

And now for the really important numbers…

64: Minutes it took me to do the race. This is almost four minutes faster than last year, and only about 80 seconds slower than my best time here. I was able to maintain a strong effort throughout the race, and I'm happy with the improvement.

218: My overall finishing place. This is about 150 places better than last year, and pretty close to my best-case scenario of under 200. Honestly, I had been somewhat concerned about my downward drift through the standings in recent years, but this year's race gave me some encouragement that someday I can compete with this crowd. It's a long-term goal of mine to make the top 100 here – and even though I got my annual whuppin' this year, I'm generally satisfied with my performance.

I've got a long time to build up to my long term goal, and I'm determined to do it. No matter how many little kids I need to knock over to get there.

Boston or Big Sur?

The third Monday in April is an important day for runners – it's the date of the Boston Marathon, the oldest, most prestigious, most historic marathon anywhere in the world. Some runners train for years to earn a chance to participate.

We've been there. Done that. Still have the t-shirts to prove it.

Like most marathoners, we would love to run Boston every year. Unfortunately, it is less than 2 weeks before the Big Sur Marathon. And it's 3,000 miles away. And we honestly feel that in many ways, Big Sur has just as much to offer.

Running in the Boston Marathon is a milestone for every serious marathoner. It is the premier marathon in the United States, and historically runners could only enter by attaining a qualifying time (variable, based on gender and age) in a previous marathon.

Although qualifying times have become more lenient in recent years, qualifying for Boston is still a great accomplishment. Today's runners also have the option of participating through various charity organizations that waive the qualifying times.

As a result, over the past 20 years Boston has grown significantly in size, from less than 2,000 runners to almost 20,000 this year. And nearly every runner goes home satisfied.

The Boston Marathon experience is incredible. Everything about the race is legendary. It is held on Patriots' Day in Massachusetts, which is a Monday holiday, meaning everyone in the city has nothing better to do than have an outdoor barbecue and cheer on the runners.

If you are a musician, imagine what playing in Carnegie Hall with the New York Philharmonic would feel like (we know, the Phil plays at Lincoln Center, but just go with it). That's how most runners feel about participating at Boston – they are performing with the best runners in the world, on the same historic course that the greatest athletes of all time have raced for over 100 years.

The course features fast downhill miles through Boston's suburbs, screaming co-eds at Wellesley College at mile 13, the challenge of Heartbreak Hill at mile 21, a Red Sox home game at Fenway Park at mile 23 (timed perfectly to finish when the first runners come into town, which allows departing baseball fans to watch the race), and thousands of screaming fans at the finish line in downtown Boston.

Two of the times Mike ran Boston, he ran beside a runner with a shirt from Lowell College, one of many colleges in the Boston area with a very vocal alumni group. The entire 26.2 miles was punctuated with fans on both sides of the road screaming "LOWELL!" over and over again. He is still plagued with occasional nightmares of thousands of people yelling "LOWELL!" in his ears.

We feel that everyone who can qualify should run absolutely run Boston at least once, just to be a part of our sport's history. But local runners shouldn't overlook what is, according to *The Ultimate Guide to Marathons*, the best marathon in North America right here in our backyard. Even *Reader's Digest* had a cover article saying if a runner were to pick one marathon in their lifetime it should be Big Sur.

Big Sur and Boston are a study in contrasts, but equally impressive. The Boston course winds through city streets and ends in the shadow of tall buildings. Big Sur stays on 2-lane coastal Highway 1 for its entire 26.2 miles, past a natural landscape that looks almost the same today as it did 100 years ago.

The Boston course is flanked by one million screaming fans virtually the entire 26 miles; the energy level is a non-stop adrenaline rush. By contrast, Big Sur's remote, rugged coastline creates periods of relative solitude, allowing quiet contemplation of the surroundings. It's more of a spiritual experience for runners amidst the glorious scenery.

Some runners try to have it all and do BOTH races. We tip our hats to them. Running two marathons within 13 days is no easy feat. Running Boston is an honor. Running Big Sur is a pleasure. They both have enormous appeal to any marathoner looking for an amazing experience. We consider ourselves very fortunate to be able to say of both of them, "Been there. Done that!"

Journey of 100 Miles

Each year, on the last weekend in June, the world's toughest endurance runners gather in the former Olympic Village of Squaw Valley, California.

Over the next 24 hours, they race each other on foot over 100 miles of the historic Western States Trail, through some of the most rugged terrain of the Sierra Nevada Mountains. They climb more than 18,000 feet, and descend more than 23,000 feet while traversing deep canyons and high ridgelines on their way towards the finish line in Auburn. It is one of the most grueling physical and psychological challenges many of them will ever face.

And this year, I (Donald) will be right there with them.

The Western States Endurance Run is the most prestigious race in the burgeoning sport of ultrarunning, which is defined as any footrace longer than the 26.2-mile marathon distance. Most ultramarathons are contested on trails instead of roads, and the most common distance is 50K (31 miles). However, the number of 100-mile races across the country has gradually increased over the past several years – and every one of these races owes its existence to the success of Western States.

If running 100 miles over unforgiving terrain through frequently ferocious weather conditions sounds crazy to you, rest assured that you're not alone. In fact, the contest was originally designed not for people, but for horses.

Western States started out as a race called the Tevis Cup, which originated when a bunch of old-time California cowboys decided to compare the toughness of their horses to legendary steeds from the days of the Pony Express. Each horse and rider who covered the 100-mile trail route in a single day and night were awarded a silver belt buckle to recognize their accomplishment.

For the first two decades of the Tevis Cup's existence, the thought of anyone travelling the 100-mile trail on foot was inconceivable. Then in 1974, a 27-year-old cowboy by the name of Gordy Ainsleigh learned that his horse was suffering from foot problems and was too lame to attempt the ride.

Ainsleigh was a bit of a maverick – so instead of dropping out of the ride, he laced up his running shoes and lined up alongside nearly 200 horses to take on the trail singlehandedly. He not only finished the course, but did so faster than the 24-hour cutoff, thereby earning himself a silver buckle.

With Ainsleigh's unfathomable effort, the 100-mile trail race was born. Today, there are no fewer than 60 such races across the United States - and while some races take place at higher altitudes, and others feature greater changes in elevation, Western States remains the crown jewel among this fanatical subset of endurance events.

Western States is unquestionably the biggest event of the year in the ultrarunning community. It's like Augusta National (without the azaleas), Daytona (without the smell of motor fuel), and Wimbledon (without the strawberries and cream) all rolled into one. What's more, it affords a select few "regular" runners - such as your author - to compete alongside the world's best.

Regardless of their ability, all of the participants who meet in Squaw Valley each year realize that they are competing at the very pinnacle of the sport, following in the footsteps of legendary champions who have gone before, while sharing the course with modern-day heroes of ultrarunning. It's an alluring combination of circumstances – to such a degree that the event struggles to manage the burden of its own popularity.

Each year, an increasing number of ultrarunners clamor to enter Western States – and each year, more and more are turned away. Because the race passes through protected wilderness areas, the US Forest Service limits the number of participants allowed on the trail on race weekend. And while rational folks would find it mind-boggling to hear that a 100-mile trail race actually has to turn people away, that's exactly what happens with this event.

Consequently, Western States uses a lottery system to select applicants for the race. A portion of the slots are reserved for the top 10 male and female finishers from the previous year's race, or runners who have unsuccessfully applied for two straight years, and a handful of sponsored athletes who are given automatic entry. Another automatic category called "pioneers" includes the now-legendary Gordy Ainsleigh, the man who started it all. Now in his sixties, he still lines up at the start line each year, and has finished the Western States course more than 20 times.

In December, the lottery "winners" – seriously, that's the word we use - are notified, and immediately spend the next six months preparing for the hardest day of running they will ever encounter. They do so with equal parts excitement and overwhelming fear, knowing the challenges that await them on race day.

A short list of potential dangers includes altitude sickness, treacherous snowpack in the high country, furnace-like temperatures in the lower canyons, waist deep river crossings, wildlife encounters (mountain lion and bear sightings are not uncommon), and ten hours of night running. That's in addition to all of the medical complications that can derail a runner on race day, which contribute to a 30-40% annual dropout rate.

There's no prize to speak of, as the race doesn't award prize money. The highest honor one can earn is a silver belt buckle, awarded to any runner who completes the course in less than 24 hours, just as Gordy Ainsleigh did on the day he decided to race the horses. Otherwise, the only reward awaiting runners at the finish line is a firm handshake, a chair to finally rest upon, and the satisfaction of accomplishing a remarkable feat.

That's not much inspiration to keep a guy running for 100 miles – so there must be something more that enables him (or her, as the case may be) to get through the most difficult stretches of the weekend. Something internal, something intangible … and something I hope to tap into over the next few months of training.

The what, when, and where of the Western States 100 are the easy parts. The why and how are harder questions to tackle. Between now and June, I'll be looking for answers on the trails of Monterey County, during one long training run after another.

When I come across something noteworthy, I'll be sure to let you know.

**Postscript: this article turned into a 10-part training diary about the Western States 100 and Donald's preparations for completing it. All of the articles are available for viewing on his website at* www.runningandrambling.com.

Leaving the Shore

[Author's note: the same year I (Donald) trained for Western States, the race was cancelled 72 hours prior to the start, in response to widespread wildfires throughout the Sierra Nevada mountains. The fires were dangerously close to the race course, and placing the racers in that kind of danger would have been grossly irresponsible.

From a training standpoint, it was a very disappointing turn of events, but over the next few weeks I regrouped my training and entered the

Headlands 100-mile trail run in Marin County. This is the report from that race, which concluded my Western States training diary, and represents my first-ever 100-mile finish.]

* * *

"The fishermen know that the sea is dangerous and the storm terrible, but they have never found these dangers sufficient reason for remaining ashore."

- Vincent Van Gogh

It's relatively easy to write about the what, where, and how of a 100-mile trail race. The difficult part is trying to describe the why.

Such as … why does anyone want to do such a thing? What's the appeal of a sporting event that takes a full day and night to complete; one that grinds your body down and tears your willpower to shreds, all for no tangible reward? And just what exactly is the point of this whole sport, anyway?

Truth be told, I was asking a lot of those same questions myself on August 9th, as I stared out into the sea from Rodeo Beach in Marin County, the start area of last weekend's Headlands 100. Over the course of the next 24 hours, I came up with some reasonable (to me, anyway) answers to the "whys" – but first, let's get the what, where, and how over with.

The short story is, I finished the race. It took 22 hours and 55 minutes of constant forward motion, up huge climbs and down treacherous descents, through the heat of day and the cold darkness of night, fighting off a handful of problems that threatened to derail me along the way. 40% of the runners who left the start line on Saturday eventually dropped out of the race; fortunately, I wasn't one of them.

(However, I can't claim that I came through all in one piece; as of this writing, I'm one toenail short, with another one that appears equally endangered. All things considered, that's not such a high price to pay for the experience I enjoyed.)

In almost every regard, the race unfolded exactly like I hoped it would. I ran the first 50 miles conservatively, enjoying the beautiful day and the company of those around me as much as possible. As the sun went down and the miles wore on, I kept a steady pace, then finished strong, even completing the last 25 miles faster than the previous 25.

My favorite memory will probably be the hours between midnight and daybreak, running through pitch blackness, fighting off fatigue and soreness, with nothing but a flashlight and headlamp to light my way. The miles were lonely and quiet, with only the occasional flickers of other runners' headlamps in the distance for company.

It reminded me of playing flashlight tag when I was a kid: dashing around bushes and down dark pathways, watching for flickers of light that revealed someone else's location, while being cautious to conceal my own position in the process. Best of all, this game continued all night long, without anyone's parents making us come in for the night just when things got exciting.

I suppose that's as good a point as any to start answering the "why" of ultrarunning – namely, it makes me feel like a kid for a while. It satisfies my sense of adventure, and indulges my inner explorer – not only in discovering the natural beauty of my surroundings, but in pushing towards the limits of my physical ability.

And just as a child experiences countless challenges and difficulties while struggling toward maturity, the most trying miles of an ultramarathon provide opportunities for personal growth. Iron is only forged by fire, and diamonds by pressure; so too is inner strength built by overcoming hardships.

There's an overwhelming cultural mentality today that difficult tasks should be avoided; that volitional discomfort is an indication of some psychological oddity. Meanwhile, ultramarathons promise exactly the opposite; the expectation is that the race will be strenuous. Your body will get battered, your spirit will get broken, and you'll question your sanity and emotional stability. (What's more – you'll pay somebody a lot of money in race fees for this to happen. If it weren't for ultrarunning, there'd be a huge boom in masochism support groups. Clearly, we *need* this sport.) It's no wonder most people think we're insane.

But here's the good part: our gain for suffering through all of this is something akin to enlightenment. We understand that our bodies and minds are capable of far more than most people ever realize; that the primary limiting factors in life's journeys are the extent to which our minds can dream, and to which we're willing to work to achieve them.

These truths we discover about ourselves are what keep us coming back for more. In that regard, ultrarunners are the fishermen leaving the shore: we're fully aware that the storms might be terrible – but the rewards we harvest by venturing into the sea are always worth the hardship.

Now, I'm the first person to admit that ultrarunning is a crazy sport. It's time consuming and physically draining and profoundly trivial in comparison to most other things in life. While I take pleasure in this activity, I'm probably not the healthiest of role models for someone to emulate. In light of that, you might wonder why I've been writing about the whole thing so much.

I guess the best way I can explain it is to say that I enjoy watching documentaries about expeditions to Mount Everest. I like seeing open heart surgeries on television. I love to watch rock climbers scale the face of El Capitan with nothing more than the gear on their bodies.

None of this implies that I have any desire to be a mountaineer or heart surgeon or rock climber - in fact, I'm 100% certain that I'll never do any of those things. But it's inspiring to know that they're possible; it gives me a sense of the amazing things that everyday people are capable of.

And trust me: guys don't come more everyday than me. I'm a regular dude with faults and weaknesses who frequently has difficulty putting matching clothes together. I don't have any special abilities; just big dreams, and a determination to work diligently towards accomplishing them.

In the final analysis, perhaps that's the lesson you can take from this series: It's OK if you don't want to be an ultrarunner - but perhaps you can try to be a hard-working dreamer sometime. If you're able to figure that part out, most other things will probably fall into place.

Thanks to all who shared this Journey of 100 Miles with me. It was a wonderful run.

Western States 100 Report

One year ago, I (Donald) wrote several articles about training for the Western States 100-Mile Endurance Run, only to have the race cancelled due to wildfires.

I never forgot about the race; if anything, my desire to participate grew even stronger during the fall and winter after the summer cancellation. The following spring, I trained my tail off, and finally toed the line the next June with the best ultrarunners in the world.

Western States took me to some unbelievable places, both physically and psychologically. Some were wondrous and exciting. Others were dark and terrifying. A few were just plain bizarre. The end result was a journey that was both humbling and empowering, discouraging yet ultimately uplifting.

The race begins in the former Olympic Village of Squaw Valley. When you're milling around the start area, rubbing elbows with the superstars of ultrarunning, seeing the Olympic rings everywhere, and gazing at the tall mountains you're about to climb, you can't help but be inspired – and more than a little bit intimidated.

Over the next 100 miles, I would complete 18,000' of climbing, and 21,000' of descent traversing one rugged canyon after another en route to the finish line in Auburn. In the two steepest and tallest canyons, temperatures reached 105 degrees on race day. Fortunately, there were river crossings at the bottom of each canyon, where I soaked in the water for several minutes in order to lower my body temperature enough to survive the heat.

The river crossings continued throughout the race – in fact, the biggest one came in the middle of the night. It's situations like this – standing waist deep in class 3 rapids of the American River at 1:30 in the morning, after running 78 miles with another 22 still to go, so fatigued that you have spasms in every muscle of your body and so sleep deprived that you start to hallucinate – that make you either fall in love with ultrarunning or realize just how crazy the sport is. Or, if you're like me, both these things happen.

During the 28 hours I was on the course, I battled blisters, muscle pains, dehydration, mild renal failure, and severe nausea. I danced on the razor's edge of medical stability, needing several minutes of observation at some mandatory health checkpoints. I was so debilitated that I could barely walk at times, and so discouraged that I wondered why I wanted to.

There's a popular saying that the person who crosses the finish line of a 100-mile race is far different than the one who starts it – and at Western States, that's especially true. The course breaks you down in every conceivable way – physically, spiritually, psychologically – and makes you question every aspect of your being. It strips you of all pretense and reveals the very nature of your soul.

It's not always the most pleasant place to be, but surviving such a gauntlet instills an unbelievable feeling of accomplishment, as well as a sense that anything is possible. All from the simple act of putting one foot in front of the other.

If all this sounds insane, believe me – this summary barely scratches the surface. There's a much more detailed account of my race experience, complete with dozens of photos that captured the day and night, on my website at www.runningandrambling.com.

Every Dog Has Its Day

One of the best illustrations of the spirit of running here on the Monterey Peninsula is the "Every Dog Has Its Day" 10K race. Similarly, one person who exemplifies the great character of our community of runners is Jim Allen, founder and director of the race. Many locals haven't even heard of the event, since it is never advertised, but several die-hard runners on the Peninsula look forward to it every January.

Jim is a retired fire department captain from Los Angeles who moved to Monterey about 17 years ago. He owned and operated a bed and breakfast in Monterey for several years before selling it and settling down.

But he never really settled down; at 67, Jim is active, vibrant, and has the outlook and energy of a 20-year-old. Running and biking keep him fit, and his optimism and joy are contagious to anyone around him.

In 1995, Jim and one of his favorite running partners, Annie, were both very fast competitive runners in local races. They frequently won age-group awards and always finished close to each other, but neither one could manage to break 40 minutes in a 10K. Although they kept training harder and harder, they could never quite dip under the elusive goal time - sometimes missing by mere seconds.

Annie and Jim share January birthdates, and in 1996, for Annie's 40th birthday, Jim decided to give her a very special gift. He searched all over the Peninsula and finally found, measured, and marked his own 10K course where Annie (and of course Jim as well) could finally break 40 minutes. The course he created is almost entirely downhill, and he named it the "Every Dog Has Its Day 10K" – now affectionately shortened to "Dog Day" by veteran racers.

Jim was knowledgeable enough to avoid a course that slopes too steeply, which creates agonizing strain on the quadriceps muscles and can cause weeks of soreness afterwards. He wanted a gradual downhill course in a scenic and rural area that didn't have a lot of traffic early in the morning. Finally, he found the perfect road in a remote region of Carmel Valley, with a point-to-point course that starts at an elevation of about 1,100 feet and finishes at 500 feet.

Jim and Annie invited about 50 of their closest running friends and had a private race. Everyone met near the finish area before dawn, and volunteers in vans and pick-ups drove everyone to the starting line. Just as the sun came up, and following his pre-race instruction to "Be careful out there," Jim yelled, "GO!" and the race was on.

Predictably, both Jim and Annie broke the magical 40-minute mark that morning. Annie ran 39 minutes and 15 seconds, and Jim surprised everyone, including himself, with a 4-minute personal best, finishing in an astounding 36:41. The runners all gathered at Jim's house after the race for a pot-luck buffet brunch and birthday celebration.

Over the next year, Jim consistently broke 40 minutes in every 10K he ran - even those that weren't all downhill. By racing on his own "Dog Day" course, he realized what it felt like, both physically and mentally, to run fast. He learned how to maintain a hard, somewhat uncomfortable effort, for an entire race. Most of all, he had a Zen-like realization that "To run fast, you have to know what it feels like to run fast."

Recently, Dog Day celebrated its 10th anniversary, and the two of us have been lucky enough to have been invited to all of them. We look forward to the competition and the fun every year. The race itself is a throwback to the early days of road racing, with no aid stations, and mile markers in chalk on the ground. At the finish line, the timer knows everybody and just writes the runner's name and time down on a clipboard. Later in the day, we celebrate fast running and good friends by eating tons of food at the buffet, and no one feels guilty.

At the post-race buffet, Jim provides unique awards to everyone: dog-bone-shaped keychain charms with each person's name already engraved. The men's race winner receives a trophy inscribed with "Best Dog in Show," while the women's winner receives one with the non-politically correct "Best Bitch in Show." Keeping with tradition, both winners are made to howl like hounds upon receiving their trophies.

The rest of us howl in appreciation of Jim for creating this special day, and for helping to make the Monterey Peninsula such a special place for running.

SPECIAL SECTIONS

THE BIG SUR INTERNATIONAL MARATHON AND HALF MARATHON

THE BIG SUR INTERNATIONAL MARATHON

"The coastline between Big Sur and Carmel features one of the most spectacular vistas anywhere in the world. The relentless hills and wind of Highway 1 make the BSIM very challenging (even by marathon standards), but most runners find that the beauty they experience is well worth the physical suffering."

"Runners who know of the strawberry station speak of it in reverential tones, like travelers journeying towards a holy shrine. Those who don't know the station is coming feel their hearts leap with joy and hope when they come across it. Afterwards many runners report that the strawberries were one of the most pleasant experiences of race day."

Hurricane Drums

It has been ten months, and I (Donald) can still hear them.

Most marathons make an honest effort to provide some sort of course entertainment for the runners - after all, it can be a very long time to stay focused - but none lend themselves as easily to inspirational accompaniment as the Big Sur International Marathon. The scenic coastline echoes the beauty of instrumental music, and there are several points along the 26.2 miles between Big Sur and Carmel where runners are encouraged by orchestras, jazz bands, bagpipes, or piano sonatas. However, none of these sounds come close to matching the impact of the Taiko drums at the base of Hurricane Point.

Japanese Taiko drums originated over 2,000 years ago as instruments of war. Their thunderous sounds were ideal for intimidating an enemy army from a distance. The drumbeats could be heard across the whole battlefield, and changes in pace or pattern were used for coordinating the movement of large numbers of soldiers. Once a battle was waged, the constant drumming above the din reassured and motivated the soldiers to continue fighting, no matter how formidable the opponent appeared.

During the Big Sur Marathon, runners hear the drums before they see them. Depending on wind conditions, the first faraway sounds are picked up about 1-2 miles before the Little Sur River Bridge, where the drummers stand on the shoulder of the road. The bridge sits 40 feet above sea level, and immediately after crossing it, the runners begin the 2.2-mile, 520-foot climb to the top of Hurricane Point. Hearing the drums in the distance, runners know they are approaching the signature climb of the race, and even experienced racers get a slight sick-in-the-stomach feeling about the challenge that lies ahead. Talk about intimidation from a distance.

The emotional dynamic changes at the base of the hill; the sound grows louder and louder, until you pass right in front of the drummers and see them pounding away relentlessly. Amidst the thunderous noise you hear shouts of encouragement from the congregating relay runners, and your heart thumps harder as you take the full measure of the daunting obstacle ahead. It's a pure fight-or-flight situation, and - assuming you don't quit the race right here - the adrenaline boost emboldens your spirit and puts some extra spring in your legs as you take your first bold strides upward.

Before too long your body begins to protest the climb, and the drummers are no longer in sight. However, you can still hear their drumbeats above the sound of your heavy breathing and the howling of the wind as you soldier ahead in the midst of your battle against the hill. I like to match the cadence of my strides to the rhythm of the background drums, as if I'm channeling the energy of the drums into my legs to maintain my turnover and steadily reach the summit.

Shortly before the summit of Hurricane Point, the actual sound of the drums diminishes, but their powerful rhythm still resonates in my mind. Even as I'm passing the grand piano at Bixby Bridge, or any of the other musicians in the last half of the course, I keep the sound of the drums as my primary motivation as fatigue sets in. I'm reassured in that as long as I can hear the drums in my head, I can keep my legs moving toward the distant finish line.

Ultimately I finish the race and finally allow the drumming in my head to cease. After a few weeks of rest I'll return to training, and eventually resume some challenging workouts. By now I've run the Big Sur Marathon so many times, and the sound of the Taiko drummers is so distinctively strong, that I'm able to conjure the sound in my head almost any time I need to. I frequently summon the drums when I'm ascending a long hill, or when I'm growing fatigued in the final stretch of a 20-mile training run.

Yet as the months drift toward the end of the year, my memory of the inspirational drumbeats of April grows slightly dimmer. But then the calendar turns to January, and I realize that it's time to shift my Big Sur training into high gear. Into February and through March, the sounds of the drums grow more prominent with each passing week. By the time April arrives, I can clearly visualize myself at the base of Hurricane Point; close enough to the drums to feel their vibrations, charging ahead against formidable odds.

The drums fill me with dread. They also fill me with strength. The drums inspire and encourage me, through the race and through the year. I can't wait to hear them again in person this April.

Scenes from a Marathon (1)

(Author's note: Each year after the Big Sur Marathon, we create an offbeat recap of the day's events – and a handful of those accounts are included in this section.)

The 20th running of the Big Sur Marathon was spectacular. Here is an insider's recap of some scenes that didn't make the mainstream press coverage of the event:

Most pleasant race-day surprise: the weather, which threatened to be miserable, became absolutely ideal for running.

Most consistently excellent performance: The Board of Directors and the volunteers created another perfect race day. They make everything seem easy, but trust us - they do an enormous amount of work to ensure the race's success.

Most worn-out one-liner that someone always thinks is clever: Year after year, somebody standing along the road in Big Sur yells "You're almost there!" or "Only 24 miles to go!" and thinks this is hysterically funny. Note to fans in Big Sur: we LOVE your support and enthusiasm, but we've heard those jokes before. Try something new next year.

Strangest shouts of encouragement: Marathon runners pass thousands of walkers who start their events at various spots on Highway 1. We thank two particular women walkers who continually yelled, "Nice buns!" to all the men who ran by – no matter what their buns looked like.

Most poignant spot on the course: It was hard to pass Bixby Bridge and not shed a tear for pianist Jonathon Lee, who serenaded the runners at that spot every year. Lee died from complications of diabetes in October of 2004. This year, his protégé, 15-year-old Miguel Martinez, played the grand piano beautifully, and we know Jonathon would have been proud.

Most obvious lie repeatedly shouted in the final miles: "You look great!" Inevitably, no matter how badly the runners are panting, moaning, limping, weaving, foaming at the mouth, listing to one side, or dragging a limb along the ground, they will hear this compliment over and over during the last miles. Carmel spectators: we *do* know that you're lying to us; we're just too exhausted to give a rebuttal. But again, thank you for your spirited encouragement.

Most likely spot to believe you are hallucinating: toward the end of mile 25, as the road gets warm and your body is drained of all remaining energy, you suddenly look up and see a group of belly dancers beckoning you onward. Sometimes you have to give them a high-five just to convince yourself they are real.

Best post-race ritual: Many runners head for the Carmel River to bathe their aching legs in cold water. However, Mary Akor and Mary Coordt, the first and second place women, apparently didn't get enough running as they skipped the river ritual and went out together for a 5-mile post-race run.

One example of bad juju: If you read our column regularly, you remember that predicting your own race time is bad juju. Well, someone who called himself "Iron Bulldog" (fantastic nickname, isn't it?) from Ann Arbor, Michigan, just turned 55 and ran the Chicago Marathon last October in 3:04. He contacted Mike through a local friend, and claimed he was going to run Big Sur in 3:01, beat Mike, and win the age division. Predictably, the Iron Bulldog finished in 3:18:51- more than 10 minutes behind Mike, who won his division. The lesson again: don't mess with juju.

Most welcome sight during mile 26: As we approached the final bridge across the Carmel River, two of Donald's young kids (ages 6 and 3) stood in the middle of the road, cheering and holding a large sign that said, "GO, DAD!" If the sight of something like that doesn't inspire you, we don't know what does.

Local heroes: Hansi Rigney of Pacific Grove ran the Boston Marathon on April 18th and finished 6th in her 60-64 division, and six days later ran Big Sur in 3:45 to finish second.

Susan Love of Carmel, who is on the marathon Board of Directors, lost her 22-year-old son B.J. in a snowboarding accident a few months ago. Susan ran the BSIM in honor of B.J. and won her 55-59 age division.

The battle-within-the-battle: Donald finished his 10th BSIM, placing 4th in his 30-34 age group in 3:03:24. Mike completed his12th BSIM, winning his age group (55-59) in 3:08:05. Since we keep track of these things, the score in head-to-head BSIM matchups is now Mike 7, Donald 1.

Congratulations to everyone who ran in Sunday's race, and to the Big Sur race committee for hosting another fantastic event!

Last Minute Big Sur Marathon Advice

Running any marathon can be fraught with danger, and The Big Sur International Marathon is no exception. Here is our last-minute advice, based on our combined 20 BSIMs.

Don't worry about the weather: You'll hear an incredible amount of talk before the race about inclement weather, but don't spend needless energy worrying about it. Really - what can you do about it? At this point, are you going to drop out because of rain? Take a hat if you think it will rain, but if the weather is bad you'll just have to face it. Remember - wind is just another part of the course. So enjoy the challenge and don't worry about it.

The morning bus ride: You may be on the bus for more than an hour getting to the start line. Go to the bathroom just before you get on the bus, and don't go crazy with the hydration on the bus ride, or you may be in discomfort and agony before the race even starts.

Also, just try to relax and don't waste too much energy in talking and babbling to your bus mates. The biggest blabbermouths on the bus are often the same ones who will be walking at mile 22. Don't be one of them.

Don't overdress: Bring warm clothes to the start, but send them away on the sweats bus before the race. Race morning can warm up pretty quickly, and after a couple of miles you may feel uncomfortable in anything other than a singlet or t-shirt. Wear a garbage bag or an old sweatshirt at the start, and discard it at an aid station early in the race. Wearing old socks on your hands is another trick that can keep your hands warm for a few miles until you toss them.

Don't do anything before or during the race that you haven't done in your training: First-time marathoners sometimes get carried away by what they hear people saying at the marathon expo, and end up doing some very strange things on marathon day. Just because some expert tells you a new race strategy, that's not a reason for you to try something you have never done before. Don't wear new shoes or clothes during the marathon. Eat the same meal before the marathon and run as you did in your last few long training runs. Don't do new things on marathon day!

Start conservatively: The first 4 miles of the marathon are the easiest on the course. They are basically flat or downhill, and your adrenaline, energy and excitement can sometimes carry you through the first several miles well ahead of your projected marathon pace. Be extra cautious and make sure your first 5 miles are about 10 seconds per mile slower than your projected average pace. For every second you are faster than your goal pace in the early miles, you will slow down by minutes during the last several miles. Be the tortoise, not the hare.

Enjoy the beauty of the course: Big Sur is NOT a personal record course. What makes this marathon magical is the fact that it's one of the most beautiful and challenging in the world. Some runners take the race so seriously that they forget to enjoy the scenery. Look at the ocean. Look at the cliffs. Look at the cows. Listen to the music. Don't get hypnotized by the line in the middle of the road. Let the beauty of the day carry you, and you'll have an unforgettable experience.

Hurricane Point is not that bad: Don't be afraid of the 520' climb to Hurricane Point; just be prepared for 2 miles of gradual uphill. Let the sound of the Taiko drummers at the base of the hill push you to the top. Don't work overly hard in climbing, but slow down your pace so that you are using the same effort you used on the flatter miles.

Be careful on the downhills: Many people try to make up time on the downhill sections of Big Sur – especially after Hurricane Point. Going too fast on the downhills tears up your quadriceps muscles and can make the last several miles very painful. Just like going up Hurricane Point, base your downhill pace on equal effort and you will naturally go at the correct speed. Don't do anything faster!

Beware the camber of the road in Carmel Highlands: The hardest part of the Big Sur Marathon is miles 21 to 24 through Carmel Highlands. You are tired. It's late in the race. It's very hilly. And the road slants a lot from one side, placing new strains on your sore feet and legs. Look for the flattest route through the Highlands, which isn't always the shortest tangent - it may be toward the middle of the road, or on the shoulder to the left. Keep your wits about you and find the best line to run.

Be ready for D-minor hill at D-major time: The last hill on the marathon is aptly named according to the musical theme of the marathon. The gentle-appearing slope from Monastery Beach to Carmel Meadows during mile 26 wouldn't be much problem earlier in the morning, but at the end of the race it is an absolute bear. Just remember that shortly after you reach the top, you can see the finish line and you are pretty much home.

Celebrate at the finish: Your picture will be taken several times along the marathon course, and at the finish line. Make sure you smile at the photographers as you cross Bixby Bridge, and when you cross the finish.

Hold your hands high in triumph and smile. You deserve it! Make your finish line picture one to cherish.

Good luck to everyone who is running on Sunday- we wish all of you a wonderful day.

Strawberries Are a Marathoner's Best Friend

It's springtime in Monterey County, which means one thing for local runners: an abundance of fresh strawberries.

OK, that's not entirely true – it also means warmer temperatures, extended daylight hours, and making final preparations for the Big Sur Marathon in April. But runners also have plenty of reasons to celebrate the local strawberry bounty.

Strawberries are one of most prominent crops of the Salinas Valley from April through September. They're a nutritional superfood for athletes, with many restorative benefits that help us with our training. And if that wasn't enough, they also play a starring role in the most beautiful marathon in North America.

Nutritional Benefits

Each serving of our local strawberries provides a full day's supply of vitamin C, and powerful antioxidant protection to help the body heal and repair. Strawberries are a rich source of phenols that help strengthen cell structures in the body and prevent cellular damage in all of the body's organ systems. Running is an activity that causes chronic microscopic damage to muscles, ligaments, and other soft tissue structures in the body; the antioxidants found in strawberries help to counteract this.

The phenol content of strawberries has also been shown to decrease the risk of heart disease and certain types of cancer – but their most remarkable medicinal quality is their ability to act as an anti-inflammatory agent.

Healing properties of strawberries include the ability to lessen activity of an enzyme called cyclo-oxygenase. This enzyme is usually referred to as COX, and is responsible for inflammation and pain, especially in people who suffer from arthritis. Strawberry phenols help inhibit production of this enzyme.

If this sounds familiar, it should: most COX inhibitors are better known by their pharmaceutical name – non-steroidal anti-inflammatory drugs (NSAIDs) – or by brand names such as Advil or Motrin. So the next time you're feeling sore after a hard workout, a tall, cold strawberry smoothie may be the perfect concoction to decrease soreness and help your muscles recover quickly. Not to mention, they taste fantastic.

Marathon Refreshment

It's a fitting combination then for Monterey County's finest crop to team up with Monterey County's finest road race, the Big Sur Marathon, on the last Sunday of April. They make a most welcome appearance at the most difficult point of the race.

Experienced Big Sur runners grow to dread one portion of the marathon above all others: miles 21-24 through Carmel Highlands, where the road rises and falls mercilessly, and when runners are in their most fragile mental and physical state. It's the stretch of road where enjoyable or successful marathons frequently go to die.

There is, however, one outpost of comfort and relief during this daunting stretch of the race: the strawberry station at mile 23. A group of Highlands residents stand among race volunteers to hand out fresh strawberries to weary runners struggling towards the finish line.

Runners who know of the strawberry station speak of it in reverential tones, like travelers journeying towards a holy shrine. Those who don't know the station is coming feel their hearts leap with joy and hope when they come across it. Afterwards many runners report that the strawberries were one of the most pleasant experiences of race day.

Of course some marathoners feel too hurried to stop for the berries. They may be wary of eating something unfamiliar or paranoid about losing precious seconds by slowing down to indulge. Or maybe they're fearful that if they stopped they might enjoy the moment so much that they'd decide to kick their feet up and stay a while.

Those runners are missing something truly special. Almost everyone who has stopped at the strawberry station considers it one of the highlights of his or her race. The thought of fresh berries in the distance helps keep them moving through the hardest miles of the race, and once they recharge their batteries with nature's superfruit they have more energy to conquer the final 5K.

Thankfully, runners who skip the aid station won't completely miss out on the strawberry bounty at Big Sur – because one of the things awaiting them at the buffet table in the finisher's tent is an enormous stack of strawberry crates. So in addition to bagels and water and energy bars, all runners leave the course with a full basket of Monterey County strawberries.

Those strawberries are always the first items we consume and they never fail to be absolutely delicious. Maybe it's the circumstances of complete exhaustion or post-race satisfaction, but those post-race strawberries are among the best things we've ever tasted.

So this spring, whether you're racing a marathon or not, be sure to incorporate this powerful little berry into your running routine. We're certain that you'll be happy with the results.

Scenes from a Marathon (2)

The 2006 Big Sur Marathon is in the books. You've read the articles telling you the primary results: who won the race, how many people finished, etc … but there's always so much more to the story. Here, then are some details that didn't make headlines, but were memorable nonetheless, from this year's event.

Cool new pre-race ritual: With his sisters at Grandma's house and his Mom out to dinner, my (Donald's) son chose to relax at home and watch *Star Wars* with me the night before his 5K race, which was very cool for two reasons:

1. When I was seven years old, my absolute favorite movie in the world was *Star Wars.* And every time I think this kid and I don't have much in common, he never fails to do something exactly the way I would have at the same age. And…
2. No matter how many times you see it, watching Luke Skywalker blow up the Death Star is simply a fantastic motivational boost. I had the *Star Wars* theme blaring in my head the next morning, and it helped carry me through some very rough patches.

Best way to start a race: I can't claim to be Scottish, but there's no more inspirational song to hear at the beginning of a marathon than "Scotland the Brave" played on the bagpipes, which has become a BSIM standard over the years. It never fails to put a bounce in your step and courage in your heart.

In fact, I've made a mental note to travel to Scotland some day, just to see what all this bravery fuss is about.

Karnazes spots the field 10 minutes: A lot of us were on the lookout for ultrarunner Dean Karnazes making his way south on Highway 1 for the first half of his out-and-back double marathon. Unfortunately, Karnazes was a bit behind schedule, leading to the unusual scene of thousands of marathoners yelling "Hi Dean!" to him during the first mile while he passed in the opposite direction, finishing his run to the start line before turning around and running an "official" time of 3:33.

This wasn't in the race brochure: On an open stretch of road during mile 7 lay a skunk that had probably met its untimely demise under the wheels of the countless buses traversing the road in the early morning darkness. The result was the aroma of freshly-killed skunk drifting almost a full mile down the course, growing increasingly strong until runners finally passed the scene of the crime.

Biggest missed opportunity: When we crested Hurricane Point, thick fog was all around us – we couldn't even see the ocean directly below. I felt bad for the runner from Indiana next to me and commented in true Yogi Berra fashion, "It's a really nice view here, when you can see it."

Then again, maybe missed opportunities are OK sometimes: Of course, when the sun did finally come out, temperatures warmed up very quickly. It went from "cool and foggy" to "hot and stifling" faster than any year that we can recall.

Most unexpected race garb: My 2-year-old daughter's favorite shirt is solid blue with a giant Cookie Monster face depicted on it; imagine my surprise to see a runner on race morning with the exact same shirt. I didn't even know they made an adult version. I wonder if you can special order it in coolmax.

Sharing the love: I ran most of the race very close behind or just ahead of the 1st place woman. Appropriately, the spectators and walkers go crazy when the first place girl runs by. I heard a full three hours worth of "Go girl!" or "Hey – first woman!" and all sorts of whooping and hollering. For some reason, the crowds don't make as big a fuss over the 28th place male. But running near the lead woman is a nice way to hear a lot of cheers – and if you close your eyes, you can just pretend they are for you.

Completely random and improbable accomplishment: This was my fourth straight year of being the 28th overall finisher. I'm not flashy, good-looking, or blazing fast, but you can call me Mr. Consistency.

The sons also run: My 7-year-old son ran the 5K, then hung around the marathon course to cheer me across the final bridge at mile 26. He then ran the rest of the way with me to the finishing chute, thereby crossing the marathon finish line ahead of Mike's 31-year-old son, who ran his first Big Sur Marathon in 3:30. Both dads were very proud.

After pain comes pleasure: There's really no way to describe how good it feels to be massaged by six hands at once shortly after finishing a marathon, but that's just what happened in the massage tent following the race. If we could figure out some way to go back several times, one of these years we might just skip the race, and duck in and out of the massage tent throughout race morning. That alone could be worth the price of a race entry.

The streak is over: Mike's Lance Armstrong-like streak of consecutive age group victories came to an end this year, as he finished second in the 55-59 age group in his slowest Big Sur Marathon time of 3:12. When it was announced at the awards ceremony, the crowd let out a collective gasp like when Mandisa was voted off *American Idol.* Count on Mike to have the eye of the tiger next year when he turns 60; all you 60-year-olds should be very afraid.

Best reason to make friends with fast relay runners: Individual age group winners traditionally receive a bottle of Blackstone Monterey County wine. The winning 5-person relay teams don't get separate bottles, but instead are awarded a large magnum bottle. You know they have to open that bottle sometime – so why not stop by with a corkscrew some night to congratulate them?

Warmest reception for age group winners: Hugo Ferlito, chairman of the BSIM board, stands on the podium while awards are handed out after the race. He shakes the hand of each winner as they exit the stage, and when local runners pass by, he embraces them in a warm hug. It's a great feeling to get a bear hug from the chairman – and just another example of the hometown charm at this world-class race.

The Big Sur Marathon for Dummies

Sometimes it's hard for non-runners to understand what all the excitement is about when it comes to marathons. Here's a primer on basic facts about the event, and this weekend's Big Sur Marathon in particular, so you can dazzle your friends with your newfound knowledge.

Q: The marathon is a long race, right?

A: Umm … yes, it's very long. The standard distance is 26.2 miles.

Q: Who came up with that number?

A: The race commemorates a victory of the Athenian Army over the invading Persians at the city of Marathon in 490 B.C. The Greeks dispatched a messenger to announce the victory back in Athens, approximately 24 miles away. The messenger, Phedippides, died from exhaustion immediately afterward. Uplifting story, huh?

Q: What about the extra 2.2 miles?

A: At the 1908 London Olympics, England's Royal Family wanted the course lengthened so that it would start in front of their residence at Windsor Castle, and finish in front of their viewing box at Olympic Stadium. The distance was changed to 26.2 miles and sanctioned as the official distance.

Consequently, it's not uncommon for exhausted marathon runners to repeatedly curse the Queen during the final two miles of the race.

Q: Do the runners get any help?

A: Definitely. Several hundred volunteers work at aid stations along the course handing out water, Gatorade, and nutritional aids to the runners. Many others provide things like traffic control and medical support throughout the event.

Q: How come on the other 364 days of the year, runners won't drink anything that isn't in a factory-sealed, tamper-resistant container, yet on marathon day they'll gladly grab unmarked open cups from any potential psychopath standing on the side of the road?

A: Good question. Maybe runners are inherently trusting. Maybe their judgment is impaired from glycogen depletion. Probably a little of both.

Q: Almost every city has a marathon. Why is Big Sur so special?

A: Easy – it's because of the course. The coastline between Big Sur and Carmel features one of the most spectacular vistas anywhere in the world. The relentless hills and wind of Highway 1 make the BSIM very challenging (even by marathon standards), but most runners find that the beauty they experience is well worth the physical suffering.

Q: Why do local runners get so geeked over this weekend?

A: Think of it this way: if you could get a group of your best friends together to play a softball game at Fenway Park, would you do it? Local runners are a close community, and our hometown marathon is one of the most prestigious in the world. The friendly competition in such a famously beautiful setting is an opportunity that's hard to pass up.

Q: Great, but I'm not a runner. Why should I care?

A: Because those people crossing the finish line at Big Sur aren't professional runners – they're everyday folks. They are your neighbors or co-workers who are giving a supreme effort on Sunday, then returning to work on Monday (OK, maybe not Monday…but probably by Tuesday) to resume their routine lives.

Many of them are fulfilling a dream by doing the marathon, and every one of them has overcome numerous challenges just to finish. Sure, by the time they reach Carmel, most of them look like hell and stink to high heaven – but each runner is a reminder that through hard work and dedication, great things can be accomplished by all of us. It's an idea that anyone can get excited about.

Good luck to everyone who is running – or watching – the race!

The Spectator's Guide to Spectating

As much as we'd like everyone to experience running the Big Sur Marathon, we realize that not everyone is able to line up with us on the last Sunday in April. We even understand that some of our readers are (gasp!) not even runners.

But that doesn't mean you can't be part of our favorite race. It's actually quite easy to be a spectator; while the runners invest several months preparing for race day, all you need to do is spend a little time learning how to be a good fan. It only takes a few minutes – by coincidence, about as long as it takes to read this column.

Spectators are an important part of the race, and the things you yell have an impact on runners. Although we might not always respond, we can definitely hear you.

Your comments and encouragement can push us forward with renewed vigor and enthusiasm – that's the good news. The bad news is, if you say the wrong thing, it may plunge us into the depths of despair. (Not to put any pressure on you or anything.)

Whether you are rooting for one particular runner, or just out watching the masses parade by for entertainment, we want to help you scream the right thing. More importantly, we want to make sure you don't screw up our race. So we've created a spectator's guide for yelling at runners.

First, understand that positioning is key. Most people like to stand within sight of the finish line to see their runners come in. But with so many people shouting, it's very hard to hear familiar voices – and honestly, at that point, it doesn't matter what you yell. By the time we've reached the finishing chute, we're pretty certain that we're going to finish – even if we have to crawl across the line.

If you want your runner to hear you, and really want to assist them, move on down the course. Shouting some encouragement with about a mile or half-mile to go can be a lifesaver at times.

Also, if you're one of the volunteers or spectators further down the course (like Carmel Highlands or Palo Colorado) with runners passing you on lonely stretches of road, you have a powerful voice! Utilize your position and make a runner's day.

(On a similar note … we're making a plea to the power walkers: We both know that Highway 1 is a beautiful, but often lonely road. There are many miles when you walkers are the only spectators to be found. So please don't hesitate to shout encouragement to runners going by. And in return, we'll try not to bump into you on our wobbly legs when passing on the right.)

Here then, are our guidelines for responsible cheering:

COMMENTS TO AVOID:

ALMOST THERE! From a runner's standpoint, this is as depressing as it is common. Here's the thing: we know how far there is to go, and we don't consider ourselves "almost there" until we see the finish line banner.

YOU'RE LOOKING GOOD! You lose all credibility by shouting this – it's the biggest lie a spectator can utter. We know that we don't look good. (Unless you happen to find sweaty, salty, smelly, drooling, glassy-eyed runners particularly sexy – in which case, feel free to drop us an e-mail sometime.)

ONLY x MILES LEFT! Where x is anything over ¼ mile. There is no such thing as "only" in a marathon when it comes to distances. No matter what the x is, we know those last x miles will probably be painful. Yes, under normal circumstances, 2 miles doesn't seem very far – but after 24 miles of running, it can seem like an eternity.

Plus, people have difficulty in estimating distances. What you think is 2 miles might actually be 2 ½ or 3. There's nothing worse than hearing, "Only two miles left!," running for about five minutes, then hearing someone else shout "Only two miles left!" Runners have nightmares about that sort of thing.

THE BEST THINGS TO YELL:

GO MIKE! GO DONALD! This happens to be our favorite one. A personal touch is always nice – so if you know a runner's name, shout it out as loud as you can. If you don't know the name, then shouting a bib number is OK. You can also yell something from their shirt like "GO Monterey!" or "GO Canada!" or "GO Team!" (For those wearing Team in Training shirts).

In fact, here's a fun game you can play: when a big group of runners approaches, just shout common names at random. There must be a Mary or Bill or Jose in there somewhere. You might give someone a nice surprise.

YOU RUNNERS ARE AWESOME! or WE ARE PROUD OF YOU! are great things to yell. They sound nice, and since you're just saying what you feel, there's no way for us to cognitively disprove it.

GREAT BUNS! We'll be honest – this took us by surprise last year when some female walkers shouted it to us as we ran past. But then we spent the whole year remembering it fondly. So obviously this is a pretty cool way to leave a positive impression.

(We know some women will be offended if this is shouted by men – but believe us, the men enjoy this kind of yelling from the women.)

BEER AND SOUP AT THE FINISH! Most runners will warm up to any mention of the comforts awaiting them at the finish line. Just don't tell them how many miles away it is.

So there you have it – now you can go out and make a difference when watching the marathon. Have fun, do some cheering, and appreciate the huge number of runners going by. They've worked hard to earn the honor of you shouting at them.

Good luck to everyone who is racing. We'll see you at the finish line.

Scenes from a Marathon (3)

The 22nd running of the Big Sur Marathon is history, and it was a fantastic morning for everyone involved. We're leaving it to the legitimate reporters to tell you about the winners, while we're reporting some "inside stories" from the middle of the pack that otherwise might have fallen through the cracks.

Here are some scenes from the 2007 Big Sur Marathon:

Test that toothpaste: About 15 minutes before the race start, one of the female elite runners was spotted vigorously brushing her teeth in the bushes on the side of the road for about 10 minutes. If she had won the race, we would have been suspicious of something besides fluoride on that brush. We'd also be trying the same thing ourselves next year.

We're all doves: Big Sur has the classiest opening ceremony of any marathon we've seen. Between the Marine Corps color guard, the bagpipe player, the benediction, and the National Anthem, it's a guaranteed goosebump situation.

They also release 26 doves, which take off and circle the canyons of Pfeiffer State Park. When they leave the box, the birds almost seem disoriented, which makes us wonder about what kind of morning they've had. Sure, everyone worries about the runners, but those doves also had to get up pretty early, and they too are facing a long journey to get back to their homes.

These are the kind of thoughts runners distract themselves with at the start line, instead of thinking about the 26 miles of road ahead. Until the gun goes off, that is.

It's nice to have big, fast friends: Our friend Andrew is over 6' tall, and blazing fast. He decided to take it easy during the first miles of the race, so Donald tucked right behind him and drafted his way to the smoothest, easiest 6-minute miles he's ever run. Andrew was also wearing an orange shirt – more on this later.

Obvious advice: During mile 5, Donald was in a pack with two other runners – one from Chicago, one from Maine. Neither one had run Big Sur before, which led to this conversation …

Chicago runner: Do either of you guys know about the course?

Maine runner: I think there are some hills. (To Donald) What do you think?

Donald: Um … yeah. It gets harder from here.

Put bib numbers on them! Near the Point Sur lighthouse, the cattle were restless. More than 100 cattle were running north and south in the large roadside pasture. When Donald came by, the cattle were headed north – at a faster pace than he was. It's not exactly encouraging to get outrun by a 700-lb heifer.

The new black? We couldn't help but notice the large amount of orange clothing this year. The men's race shirts are rust orange; the new race uniforms of Monterey's running club are orange; and we counted a ton of orange jerseys by Asics or Nike. In fact, this was a topic of conversation between us while waiting for the morning bus – Donald hates the new shirts, while Mike likes them. Does the *Herald* have a fashion columnist? We need a tiebreaking opinion on this one.

Editors are pretty smart: *Herald* sports editor Dave Kellogg ran last year's marathon, and did the 10-mile walk this year. When Mike passed him this year, Dave shouted, "The 10-mile is easier!" Observant guy, that Dave.

Convincing evidence that not very many people read our column: On Saturday, we pleaded with spectators to not yell "Almost there!" when runners went by. Sadly, we heard a ton of "Almost there!" cheers throughout the course – even as far south as Point Sur.

On the other hand ... : We also suggested that "Nice buns!" would be a great cheer, and each of us heard this several times from race walkers along the course. We may have created a monster with this one.

Take nothing for granted: At about mile 17, Donald ran alongside a friend of his who was working as a bicycle medic. They had the following conversation:

Medic: Are you doing the whole marathon?

Donald: Well ... so far I am.

Our favorite signs: At the finish line, Mike's 3-year-old grandson Jeremy held a sign that said GO on one side, and STOP on the other. He turned it from Go to Stop when Mike crossed the line.

Donald's father-in-law is a contractor. So when he saw his three kids standing on the Carmel River Bridge holding GO DADDY signs made of reinforced poster board fastened with galvanized nuts, washers, and bolts to a broomstick, with handles made of pipe insulation wrapped in electrical tape, he knew right away who helped the kids make them.

Where'd all these sharks come from? Last year, Donald ran 3:01 and won an age group award. This year, he ran 2 minutes faster, and finished 7th in the same age group. On Sunday, Mike broke the course record for 60-year-olds, but came in second to his friend Chuck MacDonald, another 60-year-old who ran six minutes faster.

The Big Sur Marathon used to be a nice small-pond event for local runners to collect some awards and feel like big fish for a day. Now it's like there's a new inlet to our little pond, and a lot of big, fast fish are swimming here from out of town and eating up our shrimp flakes.

Actually, we don't have any hard feelings about getting beaten at our favorite race – because it doesn't detract at all from the enjoyment and satisfaction we find on race day.

Congratulations to everybody who completed the marathon on Sunday. You all have reason to be very proud. Let's do it again next year!

Take Our Advice – Please!

The two of us tend to be very competitive on Big Sur Marathon day, but in the spirit of sportsmanship, we've compiled some advice for our out-of-town competitors who may be new to the Big Sur course. So if you plan on beating us, just follow these simple guidelines.

Worry a lot about the weather: The fog can be so thick you might lose your way. It might rain the entire morning. And the wind! When it's not blowing directly in your face, it can potentially blow you right off the road. There are so many conditions beyond your control; the only thing you can do is lie awake worrying about them.

Squeeze in one last run: We know you're unsure if all of your training was enough. Go reassure yourself by doing a hard workout on Saturday. Try a long run along the coast or a shorter run at race speed. Now you're ready for sure.

Enjoy a great Monterey restaurant: Take an opportunity on Saturday night to savor some world-class Monterey Peninsula dining. Make a reservation at about 10:00 PM to avoid the dinnertime crowds. Eat a heavy, fattening dinner and consume a bottle or two of our great Monterey County wine. Finish off dinner with some tiramisu, a cheese plate, a B-52 latte, and a good cigar. You're worth it!

Liven up the morning bus ride: Drink as much as you can before getting on the bus to the start. The 75-minute ride really doesn't seem that long, and school buses are a lot less bumpy than they used to be. Keep hydrating like crazy once you're in your seat. When in doubt – take another drink! Also, make sure you learn as much as possible about the person next to you on the bus. Talk incessantly and be nosy. You never know, you might find your soulmate.

Best to overdress: Don't bother with the sweats check in the morning – just wear your warmest clothes for the whole marathon. And don't believe the hype about moisture-wicking fabrics; you're better off in a cotton long sleeve shirt, sweatshirt and sweatpants. Wear a rain hat over your stocking cap, so you'll be ready for both cold and rain. Remember: fear the weather!

Experiment a lot: Just because something works for you in training doesn't mean you should stick with it on race day. Why be boring? Try something different on Sunday. Buy some fancy new clothes at the race expo and wear them in the race. Never had Sport Beans before? What better time to try them than race day! Break out those new lightweight racing flats you've been waiting to wear for the first time.

Fight for position: Line up as close to the start line as possible, so nobody gets in your way. All those people lining up behind the elites are suckers. Of course, when you're up that far, remember to…

Blast off the start line: The first 4 miles are the easiest on the course. Take advantage and cut as much time as possible off your target pace – it's like putting money in the bank! Who knows, all that adrenaline and excitement might carry you through the entire race. Run those early miles as fast as you possibly can, because the course gets hillier and harder later. Pacing yourself is for chumps.

Keep your eyes on the yellow line: Remember, your only goal is to run fast. Block out all the beautiful scenery around you – it will only distract from your task. If you want to see the ocean and cliffs and cows, come back another day and drive the road like everybody else does. Don't even listen to the music. Stay focused on the line in the middle of the road. The race is all that matters.

Hurricane Point is awful: Hurricane Point is 2 miles of horrible climbing. It's best to get it over with as quickly as possible. Charge forward and pass everyone ahead of you. All the walkers will think you're a total stud (or studette) that way. Those people won't see you later in the race, so go for it!

Run really fast on the downhills: The best way to make up time from all the uphills is to hammer the downhill sections. Regain any lost time as quickly as you can. All the minutes you lose going up Hurricane Point can be made up by flying wildly down the backside. Run like a maniac!

Embrace the camber of the road: The hardest part of the Big Sur Marathon is miles 21 to 24 through the steep hills of Carmel Highlands. Lucky for you the road starts to slant a lot in this section also. Don't bother with the flatter portions in the middle of the road – always take the most cambered part on the tangents to save a few extra seconds. Your legs will deal with it later.

Spend some time on D-minor hill at D-major time: The last hill on the course is a slope from Monastery Beach to Carmel Meadows at the beginning of mile 26. It's such a tough climb that you might as well just sit by the side of the road and cry. On the plus side, there are belly dancers there to keep you company.

Enjoy the ride to the finish: Not many people get to cross the finish line in the "Meat Wagon" – so if this happens, consider yourself one of the lucky ones! Once you're released from the medical tent, make sure you come up and thank us for our great advice.

Scenes from a Marathon (4)

Donald ran the 24th presentation of the Big Sur Marathon, while Mike did the 5K and worked at the finish line for an hour in his capacity as a race board member. Here are some observations from inside the lines and behind the scenes:

It never gets easier: No matter how many times we do this race, the 3AM wakeup call is always the hardest part of the day. You'd think we'd eventually get used to it, but we guess we're still waiting.

Are we there yet? Part 1: As soon as the course left the trees at mile 5, someone near Donald looked at the road ahead and asked, "Is that Hurricane Point?" Not yet … but keep running. You'll find it.

Most unexpected dose of hipness: was provided by the Palma High School band, overheard playing a Violent Femmes song at mile 9. Sure, the song was "Blister in the Sun", which isn't the most promising phrase for a group of marathoners, but the simple fact that they know that tune is pretty darn cool.

The beast is back: For the last couple of years, runners have been lucky to enjoy very mild breezes – but this year, the wind roared back with authority. It slowed everybody down by several minutes, and even pushed some folks around near the top of Hurricane Point. We kind of like it when the wind flexes its muscles – we don't want anybody tempted to call this race easy.

Are we there yet? Part 2: At two different points on the Hurricane Point climb, a group of runners crested a hill around a curve and shouted "Woo Hoo! Made it!", only to peer around the bend and realize that the hill keeps going. Here's how you know you're at the top: when you start leaning downhill, but you're not moving because the wind is blowing so hard. Until then, it's better not to ask.

You've heard of us? Having names on race bibs ensured that nobody was anonymous on the course. We'd like to think that the people yelling

"Go Donald!" and "Nice job, Mike!" happen to be fervent readers of our column, but we know better. The bibs were a nice touch.

If you want a lot of friends, carry balloons: there were huge swarms of people around each of the CLIF Bar pacesetters, who carried balloons indicating their estimated finish times. In between, there were long stretches of open pavement. The pacesetters did a great job bringing hordes of runners home right on their predicted pace.

Ask an obvious question ... : the most common answer by finishers when asked "How do you feel?" by Mike: "Tired!"

However, by Mike's estimate, 98% of the finishers crossed the line with a smile. We're guessing that the other 2% were happy, but just too tired to smile.

We hope your experience at this weekend's marathon was a good one. Congratulations to everyone who finished. Rest up for a while, then get training – there are only 52 weeks until we get to do it all over again!

Head for the Hills

Every winter, we receive e-mails from people looking for tips on training for the Big Sur Marathon at the end of April.

Our typical response is something like this: Run on hills. Big hills and small hills. Run every hill you can find. Steep hills and gradual hills. Run up and down hundreds and hundreds of hills. And when your legs are exhausted and you're completely sick of running on hills ... go out and run even more hills, to prepare for the final miles of the race.

The Big Sur course is a unique challenge in marathoning because of its relentless undulation. If you are training for the race, you should be heading for the hills as much as possible. But it's not only marathoners who benefit from this kind of training.

Anyone who wants to be a better runner should also incorporate hill training to his or her routine. Novice runners are sometimes apprehensive about running on hills, but any veteran racer knows that hills are the runner's best friend. So if you are a strictly flat-terrain runner, get off the straight and narrow, and spice up your running with some challenging hills.

The benefits of hill running are numerous. From a physiological standpoint, hill running burns more calories, makes your muscles stronger, and improves your body's oxygen-carrying capacity. These changes will make you faster once you return to flat terrain. Frank Shorter, gold medalist in the 1972 Olympic marathon, famously said that, "Hills are speed work in disguise."

Psychologically, hill running forges great strength of character. There's nothing like the feeling of conquering a hill that once seemed insurmountable, or reaching the summit of a long, grueling climb. And the views from the top are incredible.

Experienced runners become emotionally attached to their favorite climbs, as these hills are often the sites of their most memorable runs. In fact, many of the Monterey Peninsula's major climbs have been given distinguishing nicknames. Some are intimidating, such as Black Death, The Grind, or Hurricane Point. Others are more affectionate or descriptive, such as The Three Bears, Clara's Summit, Skyclimb, or Sky Trail .

Marathon runners sometimes ask if they can simulate hills on the treadmill. Our answer is no – because proper hill training means going both up and down the hills. Downhill running is the primary cause of soreness (and in severe cases, injuries) as the quadriceps muscles absorb the impact of your body weight plus gravity with each step. The only way to properly prepare for this is to gradually adapt your legs to increasing amounts of downhill running. This is especially important in preparation for the Big Sur Marathon, where the downhill miles are known to ruin more races than the killer climbs.

Proper technique is important. Going uphill, you want to run with an equal effort as you use on flat surfaces. This means you will naturally slow down and shorten your stride as the slope increases. Your tendency will be to lean into the hill – but be sure the lean is coming from your ankles, not from bending over at the waist.

Downhill technique is less natural. Your tendency will be to take longer strides, faster steps, and to lean backwards. But try to stay perpendicular to the downhill slope. Shorten your stride length, let your knees bend slightly on impact, and lean your body slightly forward. If you do these parts correctly, it's OK to let your step rate become faster as you are running down the hill.

Good downhill running requires thinking and adapting. That's why it takes a lot of practice.

If you are training for Big Sur, we recommend a workout of hill repeats once per week. These can be done on any hill that requires 1 to 3 minutes to climb from the bottom to the top. Start with a small number like 4 or 6, and increase the repetitions each week. Your effort up the hill should be hard, but not all out. Going down, keep an easy effort and concentrate on form. Run continuously for the entire workout.

During January and February, many local runners use a road that leads up to a community church for a weekly early morning hill workout. We call these "church repeats," and by the end of each workout we are sometimes praying for mercy. It is almost a spiritual experience.

The church used to have a sign halfway up the hill that said, "Make a Difference!" It obviously wasn't placed there for us runners, but the sentiments were very appropriate for the workout. Church Hill repeats make a significant difference in our running performance, and in our preparation for the spring marathon season.

So take our advice and head for the hills. If the workouts initially seem painful, feel free to curse at us while you're doing them. But then be sure to thank us when all that hill training helps you finish the Big Sur Marathon this April.

Scenes from a Marathon (5)

With Big Sur's 25th Anniversary in the books, we're sharing a final handful of observations from another wonderful BSIM weekend …

Hometown victory!: Even though it started as a small hometown event, the Big Sur Marathon never saw a local runner win the overall men's title – at least, not until the 25th presentation. Big congratulations to Danny Tapia of Salinas, a recent Hartnell College runner coached by Chris Zepeda. Even more impressive is that this was Danny's first marathon; it's possible that we've got a legend in the making for future editions of the race.

Coach Zepeda tried making arrangements on Saturday afternoon for Danny to ride the elite bus, a privilege that top contenders in the race are offered by the race committee. Unfortunately, the van was already full, so Danny got up early to catch the buses with the "regular" schmoes, before taking off like crazy at the starting gun. He built a big lead after 5 miles, and never looked back en route to a 90-second victory. Next year, we're guessing he'll be on the elite bus.

Fast ladies of Pacific Grove: Note that we said Danny was the first local men's winner; on the women's side, the Big Sur Marathon has had 3 local champions: Patty Selbicky in 1987, Nelly Wright in 1988, and legendary ultrarunner Ann Trason in 1989. Interestingly, all of these women were from Pacific Grove, the same town where 2008 Olympic marathoner Blake Russell currently resides. The lesson, perhaps: if you're a speedy girl looking to win the Big Sur Marathon, you should definitely consider moving to PG.

Smiling happy little people: The Just Run Kids' 3K was held in Pacific Grove for the first time on Saturday and had a record number of participants. About 3,000 kids and parents ran on a beautiful out and back course from Lovers Point. 33 schools participated, and smiling faces were everywhere. Hopefully these are the marathoners of tomorrow.

Boston to Big Sur forever!: The Boston to Big Sur Challenge was a huge success, with fantastic feedback from everybody who participated. We're happy to report that the challenge will be continued indefinitely in years to come.

Where we shamelessly take a portion of undue credit: A special shout-out goes to our running partner Carmella for completing the Boston to Big Sur Challenge, for winning the top local female award at Big Sur, and for characteristically smiling her way through both races. We've run more miles than we can count with Carmella, so we like to think that some of those mornings together contributed to her amazingly successful week of racing.

By the numbers: This year's race saw 12,000 participants in the various events, with 2,800 volunteers helping them. 365 porta-potties were picked up. 350 gallons of coffee were consumed, along with 85,000 cups of Gatorade on Highway 1. Post race, 25 kegs of beer vanished, as well as 2400 bagels, 72 gallons of soup, and 100 cases of bananas. The numbers keep getting bigger, and the race keeps getting better.

See you next year!

THE BIG SUR HALF MARATHON ON MONTEREY BAY

"No matter who you are, chances are you'll see somebody in the pack of runners who could be you. There will be runners older than you, heavier than you, leading busier lives than you. The farther back you get in the pack, the more likely you are to find somebody who has overcome significant limitations to participate in the race."

"Every novice runner has a reason for trying this race. It may be to raise money or awareness for a personal cause, to shed some extra pounds and get healthy, or to find an identity or regain control of some aspect of your life. Race day is when those ambitions are realized, so when the going gets tough, keep reminding yourself of why you started."

Half Marathon Training Guide

Local runners are privileged to have one of the most scenic and well-organized half marathons in the country right here on the Monterey Peninsula. If you are thinking of running, start your training at least 10 weeks in advance of race day. There is also an untimed, noncompetitive 10-mile walk for those who prefer enjoying the scenery at a more leisurely pace.

A half marathon offers something for every type of runner. It presents novice runners a difficult yet attainable goal to test the waters of distance running. For recreational runners, it is a good test of overall fitness and stamina that does not require the months of disciplined training that the marathon requires.

For advanced runners, it is an excellent test of their ability to perform at a high level for an extended period of time. Marathon runners use the half marathon to work on their speed and practice race pace, while 5k and 10K runners use it to build up their endurance.

Here are some basic guidelines for your half marathon preparation, whether you are a beginner just trying to complete the distance, or an experienced runner looking to improve your race time.

Novice runners

For beginners, reaching the finish line of a half marathon is something like executing your first shakedown after joining the mob: it gives you an initial measure of "street cred" within the community of distance runners. It also gives you a taste of what sort of sacrifices would be required if you want to advance within the gang. (Using the same Mafia comparison, finishing a marathon would be like scoring your first whack job).

If you are starting from scratch or from very little mileage, use the following guidelines. Try to have three consistent days of running per week, with each day having a slightly different focus.

> One day per week should be a long run that gradually increases in distance. Take whatever distance your longest recent run has been, and increase it slightly – but not by too much. For example, if your longest run has been five miles, try to do a 6-to-7 mile run at a slow, relaxed pace.

This long run should increase in distance each week, so that you have run at least 10 miles by two weeks before the race. A great rule of thumb is to add one or 1½ miles per week to your long runs until you reach this mileage.

> Pick two other days to run each week, preferably with your three total days of running separated by a rest day or cross-training day. Do your routine mileage on these days at a comfortable pace. If you feel like it, you can throw in some "striders" or gentle speed intervals of 30 seconds to one of your easier days.

Advanced runners

Although many experienced runners run more than three days per week, advanced training can still be done with only three key workouts per week, spread between rest days or light running days. The most important workouts are:

1. Long runs gradually increasing in distance every week until 2 weeks before the race. If you are currently able to run 8 miles or more, then try to ramp your long runs up to about 16 miles. This "overdistance" training is important to develop physiological efficiency that eventually translates to increased running speed.

Don't be afraid of including hills in your long runs, even though our half marathon is relatively flat. Uphill training enhances your aerobic conditioning, and downhill running strengthens your legs. In other words, hills are a runner's best friend (you know, besides having *actual* friends...).

2. One tempo run at a pace slightly faster than your race pace. These workouts are difficult and should not be too lengthy, because they are difficult to recover from afterward. Warm up with 15 minutes of slow running, and then try to run 3 miles at a pace a few seconds per mile faster than your projected race speed. These runs should gradually increase in distance also, eventually reaching up to 7 miles at tempo pace.

3. 3. One speed training workout. At the track, after warming up, run a workout of 6 x 400 meters at the fastest pace you can maintain for all of the intervals. The pace should be uncomfortable but sustainable for the duration of the interval. Jog one lap very easily for recovery between intervals. Try to build up to 10 x 400 meters two weeks before the race.

Speed work can be done on the roads as well as the track. Use a stopwatch to run hard for 90 seconds, then easy for 3 minutes. Use the same number of intervals as above.

If you want to run more days per week between these staple workouts, make sure your other runs are relatively slow and comfortable, so you have enough energy to complete the tough workouts. Don't get hung up on trying to achieve a set number of miles per week, but focus instead on the quality of the three hard days above.

Tapering

Regardless of whether you are a beginner or advanced, you need to taper your workouts down starting two weeks before the race. Tapering allows your body to recover from the training period and start to store energy reserves for the difficult effort of race day.

Tapering requires cutting back your total mileage but still completing similar workouts. Run the same number of days per week, at your regular workout pace, but for shorter distances. A general rule is to do only three-fourths of your total weekly mileage two weeks before the race, and half the total distance the last week.

Following these guidelines should enable you to have an enjoyable and rewarding Big Sur Half Marathon this fall. Sign up for the race, then get out there and train!

Triskadecathon

The half marathon is one of the most challenging and most enjoyable race distances many runners will ever experience. And yet, for many years it has suffered a reputation as the Rodney Dangerfield of road racing: it doesn't get any respect.

Despite its growing popularity, the half marathon has struggled to overcome a significant identity crisis. It doesn't have the aura of the marathon, the popularity of the 10K, or excitement of the 5K.

The marathon enjoys widespread fame and prestige. Major races like New York and Boston receive network TV coverage, and almost every regional marathon enjoys several days of newspaper coverage before and after the event. The 5K, 10K and 1500 meters are the premier distance running events at every Olympics – where the heroic efforts of Billy Mills and Steve Prefontaine become the stuff of legend, and repeat winners like Haile Gebreselassie forge their reputations as the greatest runners of all time.

Here's a quiz: who won the half marathon at the last Olympic Games? Can you name any Americans who made the Olympic team? If you couldn't think of anyone, don't worry – it's a trick question. The half marathon isn't even an Olympic event. In other words, in the vast pantheon of athletics, the half marathon ranks below badminton, fencing, and team handball.

The half marathon is the only race that is identified by comparison to another event. Nobody ever calls the 5K a "Half 10K," or the 1500 meters a "One-third 5K," yet the half marathon goes through life as a diminutive variation of its longer, better-known relative. And if that wasn't bad enough – in some parts of the country, 13.1-mile races are called "mini-marathons." No wonder the race has an inferiority complex.

Our local half marathon, the Big Sur Half Marathon on Monterey Bay, is like one of those nerdy kids in school named Reginald Archibald von Finkelstein – saddled with an unwieldy name that's almost impossible to roll off the tongue. It's also identified by the bigger race (Big Sur Marathon) it's associated with, but has to include its location in the title to remind everyone that it isn't *actually* in Big Sur.

Monterey's half marathon gets its own day, but many in other cities don't – they're forced to share a day as the undercard of a full marathon held on the same morning. If you've ever seen a race shirt from one of these events, they say MARATHON in huge letters at the top, and half marathon in much smaller font below the logo. At the expo, half marathoners feel like outcasts when picking up their bib numbers, sometimes lowering their voice subconsciously when the volunteer asks them which race they're entering.

In the large family of road races, the half marathon is the redheaded step child. If road races were the Rat Pack, it would be Joey Bishop. If you're too young to remember those guys, think of the Baldwin brothers instead: the marathon is Alec, the 5K is Stephen, the 10K is William, and the half marathon is ... that other Baldwin whose name everyone forgets.

The sad part is that the half marathon is a wonderful race. It's long enough to be a true test of aerobic endurance, but doesn't require the 4-hour training runs that are necessary prerequisites for the marathon. It's short enough to allow a strong finish over the final miles, but only if you use a smart race strategy to position yourself well in the final 5K. It's attainable enough to welcome all variety of runners, and challenging enough to seriously test the most elite runners.

Clearly, the half marathon needs a distinctive, more distinguished name. Over the past few weeks, we've been racking our brains to come up with something better – and after much consideration, we think we've finally come up with a suggestion for improvement. From now on, we're referring to the half marathon as the Triskadecathon.

That's right ... the triskadecathon. You heard it here first.

When you think about it, it makes a lot of sense. The root is Latin for the number 13, which just happens to be the number of miles in the race. It's an independent identity for an independent race. It also has a cool, slightly intimidating sound to it, which runners can say with pride when they pick up their race packets.

The word is just long enough, just Latin enough, and just obscure enough to sound serious to anyone who doesn't know what you're talking about. (This counts for a lot – if you don't believe us, try this: tell someone that you recently survived an episode of epistaxis, and watch their eyes fill with puzzlement and concern. You don't have to bother telling them it means a simple nosebleed.) If you tell your sedentary friends or family members that you're training for a triskadecathon, they'll think you're planning something pretty impressive.

The 13.1-mile race clearly deserves its own designation to set it apart from other road races – and that's what "triskadecathon" provides. It's a word that accurately reflects all of the race's positive attributes - plus, it's kind of fun to say, isn't it?

In the case of Monterey's race, it also helps to tidy up the name. This weekend's Monterey Bay Triskadecathon promises to be fantastic. The course is beautiful, the volunteer support is outstanding, and the race is a world-class event. Good luck to everyone who is participating – have a wonderful run, and hold your head high with accomplishment afterwards!

Spectator's Guide to the Half Marathon

As much as the two of us love races, we realize that running doesn't rank very high on the list of popular spectator sports.

Part of the problem is that races take place early in the morning. A typical 7AM start time automatically disqualifies at least three-quarters of the population from attending.

It's unfortunate, because large road races are excellent places to find inspiration in everyday life. In fact, many runners first become interested in the sport after volunteering or observing a friend or family member in a race.

So if you're one of those people looking for motivation to improve your fitness or shake up your daily routine, you've got a great opportunity when the Big Sur Half Marathon takes to the streets of Monterey and Pacific Grove.

And to help you get oriented, we've put together a spectator's guide for the race. Read on, slackers.

Tip #1: Wake up early

Unfortunately, this one is non-negotiable. You certainly don't need to be there for the 7AM start, but the men's winner will be done by 8:05AM, and the first woman a short time later. Most back-of-the-packers will be done before 10AM. If you take too much time to get rolling, you might miss the whole thing.

So you'll have to drag yourself out of bed earlier than usual. We know this is asking a lot. But there are several coffee shops in Monterey at your disposal. Think of it as supporting the local economy.

Besides, when you're at work on Monday and somebody asks why you look so tired, you can just say "I was up early for the half marathon" and sneak away before they ask a follow-up question. If you're clever enough, they'll never know that you weren't actually, you know, *running*.

Tip #2: Pick a convenient spot

The nice thing about watching a race is that you don't have to be at the finish area to feel the excitement of the event. It's more like a parade, in that you can set up camp anywhere you like. (Except that it starts at 7AM and there aren't any marching bands or candy throwers or Shriners on horseback. But other than that, it's *just* like a parade).

The race winds around Lake El Estero, down Alvarado Street, through the Custom House tunnel and onto Cannery Row towards Ocean View Blvd and Lighthouse Avenue in Pacific Grove.

A long out-and-back stretch from Lover's Point to Asilomar Beach allows you to see the runners twice in that area. The race's final miles are on the Coastal Recreation Trail toward the finish at Custom House Plaza.

If you live in Monterey or Pacific Grove, just enjoy the show from a spot close to home. That way, it will be easier to find a bathroom after all that coffee you've drunk to wake yourself up in the morning.

Tip #3: Watch for Olympians

Here's a hint: they'll be the small, skinny ones running in a pack way ahead of everybody else.

Reach out and offer them a high-five, and if they slap you, bottle that sweat – because you might be able to sell it on eBay someday.

Tip #4: Look for smiles

No, the Olympians won't be smiling. Neither will the small percentage of amateur runners toward the front of the pack who take the sport way too seriously.

But for the vast majority of runners, the race is a celebration. They've paid their dues with months of training. Race day is when they have fun and reap the rewards of their efforts. Many runners smile and talk to each other, and treat the event like a giant party.

Watch for the looks of pride and accomplishment on their faces. Sure, until runners reach the finish line, "pride and accomplishment" often looks a lot like "pain and suffering," but almost every person on the course will tell you they are happy to be there. Really. Trust us on this one.

And we guarantee that you'll get a LOT of high-fives from this group if you offer them.

Tip #5: Identify with somebody

No matter who you are, chances are you'll see somebody in the pack of runners who could be you. There will be runners older than you, heavier than you, leading busier lives than you. The farther back you get in the pack, the more likely you are to find somebody who has overcome significant limitations to participate in the race.

Watch them and say, "That could be me. I could be doing that." Because there's really almost no reason why you can't.

There are plenty of people and resources to help you once you set a goal for yourself and make the decision to start training. The running community loves newcomers; we're kind of cult-like in that regard. And we won't even make you get a funny haircut.

So do yourself a favor, and wake up early on half marathon weekend to watch the race and encourage all the people taking part. Who knows – maybe next time YOU will be out there in the pack, inspiring others to follow in your footsteps.

Racing the Big Sur Half Marathon

The Big Sur Half Marathon on Monterey Bay is fast approaching. If you have been training properly for the race you should be in tapering mode by now. Cut back on your mileage the week before the race and get as much rest as possible in the days before the race.

If you are a novice runner your approach to the Half should be very simple. Start easy and don't get excited into running the early miles too fast. Keep a steady pace that you can maintain for the duration. Take walking breaks if you need them, but keep moving forward, and draw energy from the crowds and your fellow runners during the final miles.

Most importantly, just have fun out there and celebrate your ability to run.

This week we're giving advice to runners with some race experience who are trying to get faster, striving for a personal best time or an age-group award. The rules are significantly different for these runners.

Have the eye of the tiger: Racing isn't always fun! There's great satisfaction afterward but the race itself should be a battle. Psych yourself up to fight adversity and discomfort for the duration of the race. Be mentally ready and don't feel intimidated.

Wear fast shoes: Monterey Bay's relatively flat course and smooth roads are ideal for using racing flats or lightweight trainers. Lighter shoes make you faster. If you use more than one pair in training, run in your lightest pair on race day.

However, do not buy a pair of racing shoes next week and race in them if they are not broken in – or you're destined for a morning of blisters and leg aches.

Warm up: If you are going fast from the gun, you need to warm your body up first. Run an easy mile before the race, then do three or four short sprints. Time your warmup so that you can jump in the starting chute about 5 minutes before race time. Don't be afraid to start closer to the front of the pack than you think you belong.

Hitch a ride: Not in a car, but in the slipstream of your competitors. Drafting off fellow runners is perfectly legal and saves significant energy if running into a headwind, which is common when heading up Ocean View Boulevard in Pacific Grove.

Pick runners who are going at a similar pace, and tuck in behind them for as long as they'll let you. In a group of 2 or 3 runners, it's proper etiquette for each person to take turns "pulling," but if you're sneaky you can usually get your competitors to do most of the work.

Don't be comfortable: If you are truly racing, it should hurt! If you feel comfortable, you probably aren't pushing hard enough. Races are for going beyond your comfort zone and giving your best effort. Remember: eye of the tiger.

Use "keys" to speed up: Your natural tendency will be to slow down, so use landmarks as periodic reminders to speed up. Mile markers, corners, or minor hills can all be used as keys to slightly accelerate the pace.

Push the envelope (but not too far): This is the hardest part of racing. You have to keep the needle at the absolute fastest speed you can maintain, but not so fast that you bonk in the last miles. Finding the optimal pace requires trial and error, and a lot of discomfort.

That's exactly what races are for. You can have a leisurely scenic run along the coastline any day; race day is for testing your limits. Remember that when the pace seems too hard.

Halfway done isn't halfway out: The course is roughly out and back, but the first mile around El Estero Lake makes it asymmetrical. If you start looking for the turnaround point at mile 6.5, you'll have a long time to wait, since the actual turnaround is at mile 7.5. But once you get there, remind yourself to…

Lower the hammer: After the turnaround, the course is almost entirely downhill or flat, and your race is more than halfway over. This is the time to crank your speed up another notch, and gut it out for as long as possible (have we already said that racing hurts?)

Fight for your place: Once you reach the rec trail at Lover's Point, the game is on. Try to improve your position as much as possible. Whenever you get passed, try to keep up with that person, and draft them if they continue to pull ahead of you. Try to pass them back further down the road.

Don't get complacent to run behind people either. Reel in as many people as possible. The last person you pass might be the place that earns you an age group medal. Some people let up a bit just before the finish line, so a well-timed kick can sometimes gain you an additional place or two.

Even if you are not interested in your overall finishing place, employing these positional tactics will help you continue to run hard when you would otherwise feel like easing off.

Have no friends: Think of everyone around you as a competitor. Get mean. Be aggressive. Breathe fire. Even if you are racing with training partners, during the race you should be enemies. There's no shame in outsprinting someone right into the finishing chute – even if that person happens to be your spouse. Give no gifts!

Obviously, racing requires an entirely different mindset than running just to complete the distance. It's definitely not for everybody. When you put so much of yourself on the line, the disappointment when you fail to reach your goals can be miserable, but the exhilaration when you succeed is sublime.

Whether you are going for an age group award, a personal record, or just trying to go the distance, we hope everyone has an enjoyable and satisfying race at the Big Sur Half-Marathon on Monterey Bay.

Acknowledgements

We would like to thank our editors at the *Monterey Herald*, Dave Kellogg and Scott Forstner, for their continuing support of The Running Life column. We are grateful for such a public platform to promote our sport, and for the *Herald*'s commitment to the health and fitness of our community.

Thank you to MediaNews Group for allowing us to reprint these columns – all but one of them, that is. One article in this collection was censored by our editors on the eve of publication, deemed unfit to appear in the *Herald*; we challenge you to identify which one was not allowed. Contact us at *runninglife@runningandrambling.com* if you'd like to guess which column was censored, or with any other feedback or questions you have about this collection.

We're grateful for permission to use the cover photo by the talented Randy Tunnell, and we're quite impressed at how he somehow managed to make us look good.

Editorial review from the iUniverse staff was invaluable, with particular thanks and appreciation to George Nedoff, Sandra Spicher, Ashleigh Wiens, and Jade Council for their help and guidance. We guarantee that any grammatical or formatting errors in this text are our fault, not theirs.

Lastly, we are especially honored by our many running friends in the Monterey Peninsula and beyond for your constant support, encouragement, and article ideas. You may not realize it, but you are all a constant source of inspiration to both our running and our writing.

About the Authors

Donald Buraglio ... is a physical therapist with more than 20 years of experience in endurance sports. He has a degree in exercise physiology from UCLA, where he was a member of the varsity rowing team. His physical therapy degree comes from the University of North Carolina.

Donald began his distance running habit while in college, and ran his first marathon at age 22. He has gone on to compete in a variety of events ranging from 1-mile track races, hundreds of road races, dozens of marathons, as well as ironman distance triathlons, ultramarathons, and 100-mile trail runs. He has competed in some of the most famous endurance events in the world, including the Boston Marathon, Pikes Peak Marathon, Wildflower Triathlon, Dipsea Race, and the Western States Endurance Run.

Donald has lived in the Monterey area for 20 years, and in addition to writing for the *Monterey Herald*, he is the author of the world-famous website Running and Rambling (www.runningandrambling.com), one of the top-ranked running blogs on the Internet. His website has won best blog, best endurance blog, and best health blog awards from reader polls of triathletes and runners. Donald is also a barefoot running aficionado, and dreams of doing an ultramarathon with naked feet someday.

When not working, running or writing, Donald enjoys spending as much time as possible with his wife and three children in Carmel Valley, California.

Michael Dove ... is retired after a 32-year career in information systems management. He also has 25 years of experience in all aspects of distance running; as a competitor, race organizer, coach, speaker, and writer. He has a BA in Economics and MBA in Finance from the University of California at Berkeley and played intercollegiate golf.

He is on the Board of Directors of the Big Sur Marathon as well as other races in the Monterey Bay area. He developed the nationally recognized and award-winning Just Run youth program and the Take 5 to Run program. He has been on the executive board of the Big Sur Distance Project and the Steps to a Healthier Monterey County project. He is also President of the local USATF running club, the Monterey Bay Wednesday Night Laundry Runners. Michael has coached hundreds of runners in marathon and half marathon training sessions and is the author of the Big Sur Marathon training manual. In 2008 he received a National Jefferson Award for Public Service for his running related volunteer activities.

As a runner, Mike competes in track and field, cross country, and road races. He has been one of the best Masters and Senior runners in the United States for the past 20 years, and has won USATF National Championships on the track and on the roads. He ran a 15:36 5K at age 49 to equal the U.S. National record. He also ran a 32:20 10K at age 52, and holds age group records in several marathons including the Big Sur Marathon.

He currently lives in Corral de Tierra with his wife, and has three grown children and 4 grandchildren. He dreams of emulating Ed Whitlock, currently the only 70-year-old who has broken three hours in the marathon.